FOOD PROCESSING
AND
NUTRITION

FOOD SCIENCE AND TECHNOLOGY

A SERIES OF MONOGRAPHS

Maynard A. Amerine, Rose Marie Pangborn, and Edward B. Roessler, PRINCIPLES OF SENSORY EVALUATION OF FOOD. 1965.

C. R. Stumbo, THERMOBACTERIOLOGY IN FOOD PROCESSING, second edition. 1973.

Gerald Reed (ed.), ENZYMES IN FOOD PROCESSING, second edition. 1975.

S. M. Herschdoerfer, QUALITY CONTROL IN THE FOOD INDUSTRY. Volume I — 1967. Volume II — 1968. Volume III — 1972.

Hans Riemann, FOOD-BORNE INFECTIONS AND INTOXICATIONS. 1969.

Irvin E. Liener, TOXIC CONSTITUENTS OF PLANT FOODSTUFFS. 1969.

Martin Glicksman, GUM TECHNOLOGY IN THE FOOD INDUSTRY. 1970.

L. A. Goldblatt, AFLATOXIN. 1970.

Maynard A. Joslyn, METHODS IN FOOD ANALYSIS, second edition. 1970.

A. C. Hulme (ed.), THE BIOCHEMISTRY OF FRUITS AND THEIR PRODUCTS. Volume 1 — 1970. Volume 2 — 1971.

G. Ohloff and A. F. Thomas, GUSTATION AND OLFACTION. 1971.

George F. Stewart and Maynard A. Amerine, INTRODUCTION TO FOOD SCIENCE AND TECHNOLOGY. 1973.

Irvin E. Liener (ed.), TOXIC CONSTITUENTS OF ANIMAL FOODSTUFFS. 1974.

Aaron M. Altschul (ed.), NEW PROTEIN FOODS: Volume 1, TECHNOLOGY, PART A — 1974. Volume 2, TECHNOLOGY, PART B — 1976.

S. A. Goldblith, L. Rey, and W. W. Rothmayr, FREEZE DRYING AND ADVANCED FOOD TECHNOLOGY. 1975.

R. B. Duckworth (ed.), WATER RELATIONS OF FOOD. 1975.

A. G. Ward and A. Courts (eds.), THE SCIENCE AND TECHNOLOGY OF GELATIN. 1976.

A. E. Bender, FOOD PROCESSING AND NUTRITION.

In preparation

John A. Troller and J. H. B. Christian, WATER ACTIVITY AND FOOD.

D. R. Osborne and P. Voogt, THE ANALYSIS OF NUTRIENTS IN FOODS.

Food Processing and Nutrition

ARNOLD E. BENDER

Department of Nutrition
Queen Elizabeth College
Campden Hill Road
London W8 7AH

1978

ACADEMIC PRESS

London · New York · San Francisco

A Subsidiary of Harcourt Brace Jovanovich, Publishers

ACADEMIC PRESS INC. (LONDON) LTD.
24/28 Oval Road
London NW1 7DX

United States Edition published by
ACADEMIC PRESS INC.
111 Fifth Avenue
New York, New York 10003

Library of Congress Catalog Card Number: 77-75370
ISBN: 0-12-086450-9

Set in Linotron Times and Univers
and printed in Great Britain
by T. & A. Constable Ltd., Edinburgh

PREFACE

The scientific literature of the effects of processing and cooking on the nutritional value of foods is not nearly as extensive as that dealing with many of the other aspects of food such as the processes themselves and the effects on other qualities. This is almost certainly a reflection of the greater interest in taste, appearance and texture than in nutritional value.

The literature that is available may sometimes appear to be contradictory but this is due to considerable differences between laboratories and factories in their raw materials and the conditions of treatment and experiment. Hence it is difficult to draw general conclusions or to forecast nutrient stability with any reliability.

There is an increasing interest in this subject largely stimulated by the introduction of Nutritional Labelling in the United States and by the growing influence of consumer groups as well as by greater interest in nutrition by manufacturers and Governments. Consequently, the rate of research in this area has accelerated in recent years.

Readers of this book may fall into two groups, those who require a general outline of the subject – and it is hoped they are adequately catered for in the text – and those who require specific and detailed information about a particular product or process. For the latter readers a fairly representative selection of the literature has been listed in a form intended to be helpful. While the text starts with the properties of the nutrients, then proceeds to processes and finally to commodities, the references start with commodities since this may be the starting question, then proceed to processes and finally nutrients. Thus a paper discussing the effects of canning on the B vitamins of meat will be listed under Meat and Meat Products and cross referenced under Canning and B Vitamins.

The references, which are not necessarily referred to in the text, are not intended to be comprehensive but to provide an entry into the literature.

Certainly modern teaching of Food Science deals with processes rather than commodities but it is suggested that this approach will be more useful in supplying the required information not only for Food Scientists but for Nutritionists, Dietitians, Agriculturalists and the many other disciplines interested in the food field.

November, 1977   Arnold E. Bender

Writing a book is a strain on the author, his typewriter and his wife, in that order. Since the references are a major feature of this book and since they were the pride and joy (!) of the author's wife for many apparently endless months, I not only thank Deborah for all she did but dedicate the book to her.

CONTENTS

Section A

Principles

Chapter 1

GENERAL PRINCIPLES

There is a general belief that when the housewife buys fresh foods and cooks them herself she retains all the nutrients, whereas when the same foods pass through the hands of the food processor those nutrients are largely if not completely destroyed. This belief is not only untrue, like so many other popular beliefs concerning nutrition, but there is no sharp distinction between home-prepared and factory-processed foods in their nutritional values. Some foods, freshly harvested and well cooked by the housewife, are nutritionally superior to those that have passed through the commercial chain, others are inferior to those manufactured under controlled conditions. Moreover, faith in the superiority of home-prepared foods rests on the belief that all mothers are good cooks, which is far from true. There is undoubtedly a large-scale, preventable, destruction of nutrients, not to mention texture and flavour, executed by vast numbers of well-intentioned mothers.

At the same time there is often a lamentable ignorance and lack of interest among food manufacturers in the science of nutrition. While it is largely true that people do not buy food for its nutritive value but for its taste, this does not absolve the manufacturer from his responsibilities.

The term 'processing' covers an enormous field of widely differing treatments carried out for a diversity of purposes; the losses that result can be grouped as follows.

1. Intentional losses, such as when cereals are milled to remove unwanted bran, or vegetables are trimmed or fish eviscerated or foodstuffs extracted from the raw material (starches, sugars, fats, protein isolates).

2. Inevitable losses, such as when food is cooked, blanched, canned, dried or sterilised.

3. Accidental and/or avoidable losses, due to inadequate control.

Whether or not such losses are a matter for concern cannot be answered as a generalisation. If there is no evident malnutrition in the community then it appears logical to conclude that the losses are of no significance. However, the earliest stages of malnutrition are extremely difficult to diagnose and there is not sufficient information available in any community to allow conclusions to be drawn about the nutritional status of the lowest end of the scale. Any reduction in nutrient intake may have some effect on some

3

sections of the community even when the average intake is well above recommended levels.

The views of the nutritionist may differ from those of the food scientist and the consumer (and the law maker). The nutritionist would view the nutritional losses from any particular food against the diet as a whole and may conclude that they are of no significance. The food scientist, however, may regard any avoidable loss as poor commercial practice. The consumer is likely to make direct comparisons between foods, whether or not the differences are significant.

Direct comparisons of factory processing with domestic cooking are rarely possible. Many factory processes include partial or even complete cooking so that factory losses simply replace those that would inevitably take place in the home.

The subject is a vast one because each nutrient, each food, each process and the same process in each factory, can produce different results. There is a large literature on the subject, some apparently contradictory because of differing experimental conditions and it is not always possible to draw firm conclusions.

A number of broad principles should be borne in mind.

Background

1. Some losses are inevitable. Processing is carried out for a variety of purposes including preservation, improvement of palatability, texture and eating properties, creation of new products, removal of inedible parts, elimination of microorganisms and destruction of toxins. Many of these processes involve the application of heat and water treatment, both of which will result in some loss of nutrients however carefully the processes are carried out.

2. While the term 'nutritional losses in food processing' is generally taken to refer to all nutrients, the most sensitive by far are vitamin C and to a lesser extent B_1 – the other nutrients are much more stable and very little is lost in most processes.

3. Manufacturing and processing losses, where they do occur, are often in place of, rather than in addition to, those that inevitably accompany cooking in the home. For example, canned foods have already been cooked during the process and require only heating, or may even be eaten without any further preparation; many dried foods and frozen fruits and vegetables have been blanched as the first stage of the process and need less final cooking than the corresponding fresh food.

As shown in Tables 1.1 and 1.2 there is little difference between the vitamin C contents of fresh, freeze-dried and frozen garden peas after cooking. This is largely because fresh peas needed 10 min boiling, compared with 3.5 min for frozen peas and 2 min for freeze-dried peas.

Tables 1.1 and 1.2 also show that after cooking air-dried and canned peas are lower in vitamin C content than the three other samples – the former suffered a large cooking loss and the latter suffered a larger processing loss.

TABLE 1.1. Peas: percentage loss of vitamin C after stages of processing (after Mapson, 1956 [677])

Fresh	Frozen		Canned		Air-dried		Freeze-dried	
–	Blanching	25	Blanching	30	Blanching	25	Blanching	25
–	Freezing	25	Canning	37	Drying	55	Drying	30
–	Thawing	29						
Cooking 56	Cooking	61	Heating	64	Cooking	75	Cooking	65

TABLE 1.2. Vitamin C content of garden peas after processing and cooking (Robertson and Sissons, 1966 [462])

Process	Fresh Variety 1	Variety 2	Frozen	Freeze-dried	Air-dried[a]	Canned[b]
Time boiled (min)	10	10	3.5	2	15	brought to boil
Vol. water (×vol. food)	1.2	1.2	1	12.3	23.6	–
Vitamin C (mg/100 g)	16.4	18.5	14.0	15.8	11.3	9.2

[a] large cooking loss; [b] large processing loss.

Similarly Abrams (1975) [308] showed that fresh sprouts required 20 min cooking and lost 36% of the vitamin C, while the frozen ones required only 10 min cooking and lost a total of 41% of the vitamin.

4. Where losses of nutrients take place the relative importance of the food in question as a source of the particular nutrient must be taken into account. Losses from the poorer sources of the nutrient in question are of little significance (Tables 1.3 and 1.4).

It has been shown [98] that the meat of broiler chickens contains less vitamin B_1 than does the meat of free-range chickens, but since chicken meat supplies less than 1 per cent of the vitamin B_1 of the average British diet such a difference has no importance.

The vitamin C of milk is largely destroyed during pasteurisation but milk, even if consumed untreated, is not an important source of this vitamin (although it could be for some people, (see 5). On the other hand, although potatoes are not a rich source of vitamin C the amount eaten, for example in Western Europe makes them the most important single source of this vitamin in the average diet.

5. Regard must be paid to sections of the community who may be relying to a large extent on a small number of foods as a source of nutrients. Babies may be obtaining their entire supply of nutrients from a single manufactured food, and elderly persons often restrict their diet to few items so that loss

TABLE 1.3. Percentage of total nutrient intake supplied by various foods (U.S. Department of Agriculture, 1974; U.K. Household Food Consumption and Expenditure, 1973)

				Vitamins				
	Protein	Calcium	Iron	A	B_1	B_2	Niacin equivalent	C
United States								
All meats	42		29	22	28	25	46	
Dairy products (excl. butter)	23	76		13		41		
Potatoes								18
Cereals	18		28*		36*	17*	24*	
Great Britain								
All meats	28		28	25	19	21	35	
Liquid milk	17.5	46		12	14	34	12	
Potatoes				11				26
Cereals	26	24*	31*		39*	12	19*	
Butter and margarine				26*	(46% vit. D)			

* enriched.

which may be of little importance in the average mixed diet may become a matter of importance to them.

Some of our own surveys have brought to light elderly persons and young active students who consume no fruits or vegetables (even potatoes) and appear to be getting their minimum daily needs of vitamin C from such normally disregarded sources as milk, jams and processed meats.

6. When discussing losses (and benefits are often involved) the comparison is often made between foods taken straight from the soil or the pasture and those that have been processed and stored for months. It is much more difficult to compare 'fresh' vegetables that have spent ten days in transport, in store and on the shelf with 'processed' vegetables that were frozen within the hour of cropping. Fish similarly may be considered 'fresh' when it is raw

but three weeks dead, and 'processed' when it was frozen or even cooked and frozen at sea within a few hours of catching.

Daniels (1974) [891] drew attention to the difference between 'garden fresh' (meaning immediately after harvest) and 'market fresh'. He analysed the vitamin C content and expressed the results as a percentage of figures quoted in the U.S. Food Composition Tables ($\pm$ Standard deviation): garden fresh peas 121 ± 35; market fresh 65 ± 26; frozen peas 98 ± 46; canned vegetables 102 ± 22. He concluded that frozen vegetables were similar in vitamin C content to 'market fresh'.

7. Beneficial effects. Although the effects of processing are generally discussed in terms of loss of nutrients there are many examples where the

TABLE 1.4. Percentage of recommended daily intake of nutrients
provided in 100 g food

Vitamin C (FAO figure of 30 mg)		Riboflavin	
Pears	10%	Cabbage	2%
Apples	15%	Carrots	3%
Potatoes	35-70%	Peas	7%
Peas	100%	Mushrooms	20%
Oranges	200%		
Thiamin		Carotene	
Sprouts	5%	Cabbage	15%
Potatoes	5-10%	Peas	15%
Cauliflower	10%	Sprouts	20%
Peas	25%	Broccoli	100%
		Carrots	100-200%

reverse is true. Quite apart from enrichment, which is often included among the processes, there can be a significant increase in nutrient availability. Some protein foods, and this is particularly true of legumes, contain substances that inhibit the digestive enzymes so that in the raw state they have a biological value less than their amino acid pattern indicates. Heat processing destroys these trypsin inhibitors and increases the biological value. Vitamins, and this relates particularly to niacin, may be present in a bound form, biologically unavailable until the food has been subjected to heat. The destruction of toxins is another example of the beneficial effects of processing. The subject is dealt with in chapter 2.

8. Losses must be balanced against advantages. While it is true that there are often unnecessary losses of nutrients due to poorly controlled processing, there may well be losses even under the best conditions and these are presumably the price that is willingly paid for the advantages, of which there are many examples. (i) There are losses of vitamins C, B_1 and B_2 in the pasteurisation of milk but this is regarded as a price worth paying for

safety. (*ii*) Sausages are sometimes preserved with sulphur dioxide and the thiamin is largely destroyed. If the preservative were not used there would need to be more frequent delivery to retail outlets and a consequent increase in price. (*iii*) It is convenient for catering institutions and restaurants, not to mention the housewife, to have potatoes delivered ready-peeled and ready-chipped; and to prevent enzymic browning they are preserved with sulphur dioxide. The partial destruction of thiamin may be of some significance since potatoes supply 15% of the thiamin of the average British diet. This may be a case where the price of convenience is too high. (*iv*) The Maillard reaction (chapter 4) serves as an example of a small nutritional loss in return for the desirable flavours produced in foods like roasted meat, crust of bread and biscuits. The price is some loss of available lysine.

9. Inadequate methods of assessing nutritive value can lead to false conclusions. For example, biological measures of protein quality will show a fall only when the limiting amino acid is affected; changes in other amino acids are not revealed by these methods. For example milk, meat and fish are limited by methionine plus cystine and contain a relative surplus of lysine. If the amount of available lysine is reduced there will be no change in the biological measure until the damage is severe enough to make lysine limiting. Similarly, as discussed later, inadequate methods of assay of vitamins can lead to incorrect conclusions.

10. Finally, it is not always a choice between fresh, unprocessed food with its full complement of nutrients and a processed (or cooked) food with varying degrees of damage but often a choice between canned, frozen, dried and sterilised foods versus none at all. Fresh foods are available for a limited period of time and if they are not preserved they cannot be transported or stored. In Great Britain for example, fresh garden peas are available for only about 2 months of the year so for 10 months the comparison is not between fresh and processed peas but between processed peas and none at all.

Variable composition

Plant foods can vary greatly in their nutrient content depending on factors such as variety, soil, fertiliser – type, amount and time of application – size, degree of maturity, season, length of day, light intensity, temperature, etc. The composition of animal foods is more consistent so far as the major components are concerned but micronutrients can vary. The amounts of iron and vitamin A stored in the tissues depend to a great extent on the diet of the animals and consequently on the conditions of husbandry. The composition of milk is affected by diet, management, stage of lactation, breed, exposure to sunshine, age, etc.

The handling of the food after harvesting or killing can also affect nutrient content. This applies particularly to the vitamin C in plant foods and it must be taken into account when results from different factories, laboratories or production batches are being compared.

The differing amounts of nutrients found naturally in foods are exemplified by the following list [895]: five-fold range in vitamin C in tomatoes (leading to a fifteen-fold range in freshly pressed tomato juice); twenty-fold range in 28 varieties of mango; thirty-five-fold range in 7 varieties of muscatine grapes.

While vitamin C is notorious for its wide range of variation other vitamins also vary. e.g. carotene in carrots covered a twelve-fold range and in sweet potatoes varied form zero to 7 mg per cent; there was a three and a half-fold range of niacin in 46 strains of sweet corn, and a six-fold range of linoleic acid in four sources of safflower oil.

Nitrogen fertilisers usually affect yield rather than composition but they do cause some changes. They increase the amount of protein in many cereals but because of a differential increase in some of the proteins there is a fall in quality (in aggregate there is an overall gain). For example, fertilisation of maize can increase the protein content from 7.8 to 10.4% of the weight of the food but this is largely due to an increase in zein which reduces the *proportion* of lysine from 3 to 2.4% (of the protein) and of tryptophan from 1.8 to 1%.

Nitrogenous fertilisers produce differing effects on vitamin C. The general pattern is that fertilisers increase the vitamin C in apples but reduce the amount in tomatoes and strawberries due to increased leaf growth causing shading. Size can sometimes affect nutritional content, particularly of vitamin C.

Although large-scale manufacture results in the blending of vast numbers of samples of the food in question there can still be variations in the finished product. An example of this was given by Farrow *et al.* (1973) [555] who measured the vitamin C content of canned tomato juice over an eleven year period; approximately 30 samples were analysed each year. The average values each year ranged only from 16 to 13 mg per 100 ml but the maximum and minimum values covered a wider range.

It is obvious that discarding any part of the original material such as the trimming of vegetables or meat or fish, must result in some loss of nutritive value but such losses can be disproportionate. For example, the outer dark green leaves of vegetables like cabbage contain a greater concentration of carotene and vitamin K than the inner leaves while the outer leaves of sprouts contain slightly *less* vitamin C than the inner part [308]. There is a higher concentration of some of the vitamins in the outer layers of some fruits and vegetables so that peeling results in proportionally greater loss (Table 1.5).

In preparing fish, e.g. salmon for canning, heads, tails, viscera and eggs are discarded. The viscera contain proportionately more vitamins than the flesh and the eggs are a source of protein so that the losses are greater than the discarded weight of fish might indicate. Even if the trimmings are used for animal feed it is still a loss of food intended for human consumption.

Table 1.5. Distribution of vitamin C in tissues of fruits and vegetables (mg/100 g) (from Holman, 1956 [674])

Apples	
Bramley seedlings	peel 50
	cortex 14
Cox's orange pippin	peel 10
	cortex 1
Oranges	flavedo 220
	albedo 70
	juice 50
Peaches	skin 15-40
	pulp 6-15
Pears	peel 7
	cortex 3
Strawberries	cortex 110
	medulla 70
Asparagus	tips 83
	middle stem 38
	white stem 17
Beans, runner	seeds 50
	pods 29
Cabbage	outer green leaves 90
	curled green leaves 70
	white leaves 45
	heart leaves 80
Potato	skin 10
	epidermis 13
	middle 13
Spinach	leaves 30-60
	stems 10-16

The enormous variability both in raw material and in the effects of processing is well illustrated by the work of Marchesini *et al.*, (1975) [442].

Green beans were trimmed, blanched for 1 min at 95°C, cooled, canned and sterilised either at 124°C for 8 min or 116°C for 25 min.

First, despite the fact that the samples were closely related (cultivars) and grown under the same experimental conditions the range of ascorbic acid (AA) was very great, 11 to 27 mg/100 g, mean 17.0±S.D. 5.0. Dehydroascorbic acid (DHA) varied even more, range 2-11 mg, mean 6.5 ± 2.0. Total vitamin C was between 14 and 35 mg/100 g.

Table 1.6 shows mean values for all 15 cultivars and separate figures for two examples.

Cultivar 1 lost virtually all its ascorbic acid at 124°C both from the drained beans and the brine and about three quarters of the dehydro form. At the lower temperature (but longer time) half the AA and one quarter of the DHA were lost.

Cultivar 9, however, lost only a quarter of the AA and a quarter of the DHA at 124°C and so exhibited much greater stability of both forms of the vitamin. At the lower temperature of 116°C this cultivar lost *more* AA, half

TABLE 1.6. Vitamin C in green beans mg/100 g (from Marchesini *et al.*, 1975 [442], figures rounded off)

	Ascorbic acid			Dehydroascorbic acid		
	Fresh	Drained beans	Brine	Fresh	Drained beans	Brine
8 min at 124°C						
Cultivar 1	14.0	0	0.9	7.0	2	0.5
Cultivar 9	11.0	5.0	4.0	5.6	3.4	1.0
Mean of 15 cultivars	17.0 ± 5.0	2.5 ± 1.6	3.7 ± 2.2	6.5 ± 2.0	2.8 ± 1.2	1.9 ± 1.1
Loss		84%	77%		54%	67%
25 min at 116°C						
Cultivar 1	14.0	3.9	3.8	7.0	3.1	2.8
Cultivar 9	11.0	3.4	2.1	5.6	2.1	2.1
Mean	17.0 ± 5.0	3.4 ± 1.6	4.1 ± 2.3	6.5 ± 2.0	2.6 ± 1.3	1.8 ± 1.0
Loss		79%	75%		56%	71%

compared with a quarter, but less DHA, about one-fifth (compared with a quarter as the higher temperature).

Taking the mean results of all 15 cultivars there was no significant difference between the two temperatures.

Table 1.6 shows the average results for loss of AA and DHA and the amount extracted into the brine. If 15 cultivars grown under controlled experimental conditions can show such variation it would seem to be impossible to achieve consistency of results in commercial practice.

These results apply to the canned beans a few days after canning. Vitamin C was also measured after 6 months storage. DHA had almost completely disappeared and the AA had risen by about 15%; overall there was a fall in vitamin C.

The total effect was 75% loss of vitamin C on canning with a further small fall after 6 months giving a total loss of 80%.

It will be noted that the vitamin distributed itself between the beans and the brine, so if the brine were discarded the loss would be approximately doubled.

Reliability of results

Many authors find significance in differences of a few per cent in the vitamin content of foods and quote such figures as indicative of loss. It may at the same time be noted that some authors find an apparent gain in vitamins during processing and storage. Rarely are enough samples analysed to allow statistical examination of the significance of the findings. The literature must be considered with care.

It must be borne in mind that vitamin assays are far from precise and differences of a few per cent are probably not significant. For example 4 vitamins were assayed in a variety of manufactured milk preparations in two laboratories [171]; in some samples duplicated estimations of folic acid agreed exactly, in others the variations were 0.21 and 0.25, and 1.12 and 0.91. For thiamin, again some samples showed exact agreement, the duplicates in other samples were 4.2 and 5.9, 2.4 and 3.3, 4.8 and 6.1, 8.9 and 11.6, 9.7 and 13.0. For vitamin B_6, some duplicates agreed well, others were 3.3 and 4.3, 3.6 and 4.9, 9.9 and 14.6, 7.5 and 11.9.

One group of authors [101] reported that in pork aged for 3 days and then stored at $-18°C$ thiamin was the least stable vitamin – losses increased to 33% after 24 weeks storage. The results quoted after 8, 16, 24, 32, 40 and 48 weeks respectively were, 19%, 26%, 33%, 24%, 29% and 21%. Thus the loss after 48 weeks was *the same* as the loss after 8 weeks; it seems that after 8 weeks the thiamin is stable contrary to the conclusions drawn by the authors from their own work.

A similar criticism must be levelled at biological measurements of protein quality. It is not possible to detect small differences in protein quality by any biological method since the variation between experimental results is usually at least 5-10%. Greater differences can be expected between different laboratories. Even chemical analysis of amino acids is probably not reproducible to better than $\pm 5\%$ – again many authors do not provide limits of the accuracy of their methods.

Consequently reported losses of less than 10% may have little significance both in the statistical and general sense of the word.

A further problem arises from variations between samples of food processed or stored under apparently identical conditions. Bender (1958) [313] showed that there was a range from 44 to 31% loss of vitamin C in 4 bottles of fruit squash stored under identical conditions, and differences such as 16 and 24%, and 33 and 50% between pairs of bottles stored under identical conditions. These differences were not due to losses during bottling nor to leaking seals.

Similar variations between bottles of fruits stored under identical conditions have been reported [313] – 5 bottles of blackcurrants showed a range of 28 to 43% loss of vitamin C after 16 months storage and 5 bottles of strawberries ranged between 47 and 89% loss. Harris and von Loesecke [895] make the same point when they state that published data on thiamin stability in specified canned foods show variations from pack to pack.

An obvious problem arises from the impossibility, in many instances, of analysing the same sample before and after processing and storage. All that can be done is to analyse a number of samples of the raw food and a different set of samples after treatment, and then to apply a statistical test to the significance of any differences found.

The three problems mentioned, namely, imprecision of assays, variations between apparently identical samples and the fact that the same sample cannot be analysed before and after processing, could account for a large part of the differences reported from different laboratories.

Increases in vitamin content after processing

As described in chapter 2 it is possible to liberate bound forms of certain vitamins so that there can be a true increase in nutritive value. However, some increases reported in the literature are clearly due to errors in the method although this is not always realised by the authors themselves. Lehrer *et al.* (1952) [53] reported a two and a half-fold increase in the niacin content of lamb stored at −18°C for 6 months and suggested that the vitamin was being synthesised during storage. Schweigert and Lushbough (in Harris and von Loesecke [895]) reviewing its work suggest, instead, that the results indicate 'analytical difficulties'.

In some instances the apparent increase is due to the greater difficulty of extracting the nutrient from the raw material compared with the processed food. This is particularly true of carotenoids in leafy vegetables where increases of 200 to 400% have been shown to follow heat processing. There may be some enzymic destruction of the carotene during the extraction from the raw food (which would not take place in the heated food) but the greater part of the apparent gain is due to the incompleteness of the extraction from the starting material. Nutting *et al.* (1970) [369] explained an apparent increase in the carotenoid content of parsley in this way.

Another reason for apparent gain is interference in the assay. Thomas and Calloway (1961) [547] repeatedly found an increase in riboflavin after processing. The authors explained their results either by release of a bound form (which would, indeed be an increase) or due to the development of fluorescent substances that interfere with the assay.

It is possible for B vitamins to be synthesised by bacteria growing on putrefying food. For example, the riboflavin in pork stored 14 days at 104°C was 104% of its initial value i.e. no change. After 28 days the riboflavin content had risen to 154%, and after 56 days, when the food was badly decomposed, to 141% of the initial value [81, 82].

Calculation of nutrient losses

Murphy *et al.* (1975) [912] drew attention to the different methods of calculating nutrient losses which sometimes produce quite different results. They define apparent retention as

$$\frac{\text{nutrient content per g cooked food}}{\text{nutrient content per g raw food}} \text{(dry wt)} \times 100$$

while true retention is:

$$\frac{\text{nutrient content per g cooked food} \times \text{g food after cooking}}{\text{nutrient content per g raw food} \times \text{g food before cooking}} \times 100$$

They pointed out that several types of changes occur:

Type 1. Moisture loss only. Example: Vegetables cooked by steaming.
Type 2. Moisture gain only. Example: Rice cooked so all the water is absorbed.
Type 3. Solids lost but moisture gained. Example: Dry legumes cooked in water.
Type 4. Moisture and solids both lost. Example: Organ meats cooked in water.
Type 5. Moisture and solids lost from more than one tissue. Example: Roasted poultry, which contains lean muscle, skin, and sometimes depot fat.
Type 6. Moisture lost and fat or other solids gained. Example: Fried breaded fish.

In some examples the differences are small. Thus Type 1 above applied to a number of vegetables where retention was essentially complete, 13 nutrients were measured in 6 lots of oven-roasted peanuts and although some differences were statistically significant, they were very small, e.g. iron retention 98% true vs 101% apparent.

Brown rice provided an example of Type 2; protein retention 105% true, 101% apparent.

Thirty legumes provided example of Type 3; for protein, true value 96%, apparent 103%, ash, true 80%, apparent 86%; iron, true 111%, apparent 120%.

Greater differences were found in Type 4, using simmered turkey livers as the food; protein, true 85% vs 103%; fat 107% vs 131%; thiamin 58% vs 70%; riboflavin 47% vs 57%; niacin 43% vs 53%; cholesterol 92% vs 112%; retinol 51% vs 62%.

Type 5 was exemplified by turkey meat and skin where losses from the two tissues differed (roasted until temperature rose to 145°C, internally 85°C, time not given); protein, true retention 101% vs 105%; fat 90% vs 94%; thiamin 68% vs 71%; riboflavin 83% vs 90%; niacin 92% vs 96%; iron 97% vs 101%. (No examples of Type 6 were given.)

Clegg (1974) [577] showed that loss of vitamin C from Brussels sprouts during blanching was 30% when calculated on the wet weight (which is the important measure from the consumer's point of view) but that this was due to increased water content and that the loss calculated on dry weight was only 10%.

It must be borne in mind that almost all reports in the literature of changes in processing are based on controlled processing whereas in practice many bizarre and uncontrolled operations are carried out. Hence there may be a considerable difference between nutritional changes that can occur and those that do occur. For example the literature has little application to an operation where minced meat was boiled in a large volume of water for 90 min and the aqueous fraction discarded. Such an operation was witnessed in institutional feeding and there is no evidence to suggest that this was unique.

Earlier literature

Three developments over the years may invalidate older figures reported in the literature: (1) changes in varieties of plants and growing conditions, (2) changes in methods of processing, and (3) improved methods of assay.

Examples of changes in methods of processing include the Chorleywood process for bread, the introduction of blanching before drying or freezing, the use or non-use of sulphite in blanching water, the addition of vitamin C as a reducing agent.

Varieties of food crops and strains of animals have also changed. However the U.S. Canning Industry carried out a nationwide survey of the nutritional content of canned foods in 1940-43 and found no marked change 30 years later despite changes both in varieties of foods and in processing methods [555, 568].

The values found for vitamins A, C, thiamin, riboflavin, niacin and minerals, protein, fat and carbohydrate agreed very well with those reported in the 1963 Handbook No. 8 (Watt, B. K. and Merrill, A. C. Composition of Foods. U.S. Dept. of Agriculture) – all values were within 5% except for vitamin C which was within 10%.

The carotene content of tomato juice was 850 i.u. (255 μg) per 100 g in the 1940 measurements and 647 i.u. (190 μg) in 1969. Niacin was 0.83 mg per 100 g in the earlier measurements and 1.04 in the later series. Vitamin C in tomato juice was 14.3 and 13.4 mg per 100 g respectively.

Methods of assaying vitamin C produce low results when dehydroascorbic acid is excluded or high results if interfering substances are included. Earlier evidence that carotenes were not affected in canning was incorrect since only total carotenoids were determined and it was not known that isomerisation occurred with consequent loss of biological potency. Measurements of total protein or total amino acids do not always provide evidence of change in nutritional value and the loss of some nutrients such as trace elements or polyunsaturated fatty acids may not have been of interest to earlier investigators.

Use of food composition tables

Since the composition of fresh foods varies so greatly and that of processed foods even more it may be questioned whether tables of average food composition are of any use.

First, it must be emphasised that such figures are not merely averages but selected values intended to represent the food in question. Secondly, the greater problems of variation apply to vitamins, and to a lesser extent to mineral salts, while the protein, fat and carbohydrate (and consequently energy content) of foods vary much less.

Thirdly, food composition tables are mostly used to assess the food values of total diets and to plan supplies of the major, and less variable, nutrients. Some foodstuffs such as sugar, butter and fats are both homogeneous and constant in composition, others like bread and milk are nearly so. So the table figures do apply fairly precisely to this part of the diet. Foods such as meat and made-up dishes are neither homogenous nor constant in composition. Overall it is estimated that the use of tables gives values within ±7% of analysed values – but not for vitamins and minerals.

Most composition tables provide information for cooked as well as raw foods and while there is not likely to be any changes in fats and carbohydrates (apart from addition of fat in frying processes) no allowances are made for changes in protein quality. The newer tables will at least contain information of amino acid composition and available lysine [919].

It is usual to allow 50% for the loss of vitamin C from root vegetables in cooking and 75% from leafy vegetables but from the evidence available such figures can be only a vague guide. When figures for labile nutrients are needed it is essential to carry out analyses.

The methods of compiling and using composition tables are reviewed by Murphy *et al.* (1973) [913] and Southgate (1974) [919].

Rounding off

With all the errors involved in sampling and assaying of nutrients, particularly vitamins and protein, there cannot be a high degree of precision. Some authors are clearly at fault when they quote far too many significant figures in their results such as those who quoted losses from rice stored for $2\frac{1}{2}$ years as 29.40% thiamin, 5.44% riboflavin and 3.77% niacin!

In this volume the author has taken the liberty of rounding off most of the figures quoted in the original papers. Thus the above figures would be given as 30%, 5% and 5% respectively. Losses of 5 to 10% are regarded by the writer (even if not by the original authors) as indicative of no change unless there is clear evidence of the significance of such a change. For example, niacin in pork stored for 14 days was 90% of the original, and after 56 days was 93% [81, 82]. Such values have been interpreted in the present book as indicative of no change.

Chapter 2

BENEFICIAL EFFECTS OF FOOD PROCESSING

Much of the discussion of nutritional changes in food processing revolves around losses but there are sometimes nutritional gains. Quite apart from the preservation of nutrients and food enrichment there are processes that directly enhance nutritional value. The two most important examples are proteins and niacin.

Legumes

Most legumes contain a number of toxins and substances that inhibit digestive enzymes – Liener [437, 438, 439] described five trypsin inhibitors in raw soybeans. Destruction of these increases the nutritional value of the proteins. The thermostability of anti-proteolytic factors varies with the type of food; some of those in soya are very heat labile, but there are protein-bound inhibitors that are more stable; those in wheat flour are labile, in field bean they are moderately labile, and they are very stable in Lima beans [470] and green gram [425].

Heat treatment beyond that needed to destroy these toxins causes a reduction in nutritive value (as discussed in chapter 4) and a considerable amount of work has been carried out to determine the optimum conditions [441, 472, 432]. Available lysine serves as a useful indicator of quality in overheated samples and the presence of trypsin inhibitor or of the enzyme urease is an index of inadequate heat treatment.

Other toxins found in legumes include goitrogens and substances that agglutinate the red blood cells (phytohaemagglutinins) and can lead to the death of animals fed beans such as *Phaseolus vulgaris* in the raw state. There are also substances that interfere with the absorption of minerals and vitamins e.g. zinc, manganese, copper and iron and vitamins B_6, D and E.

For example raw kidney beans have been shown to cause nutritional muscular dystrophy in pregnant ewes [742] due to a heat-labile vitamin E antagonist. Similarly *Pisum sativum* decreased the effectiveness of vitamin E in the prevention of foetal resorption in the rat.

Favism is caused in genetically susceptible individuals by the nucleoside vicine found in the broad bean (*Vicia faba*) and results in haemolytic

19

anaemia. Lathyrism is caused by an amino acid (oxalyl-diamino caproic acid) in *Lathyrus sativus*. Cottonseed meal contains gossypol which is both toxic and combines with lysine so reducing the nutritional value of the protein; it can be removed by processing [414]. Certain cruciferous oilseeds such as rape and mustard contain goitrogens (allyl isothiocyanate and vinyl-oxazolidine thionine). Lima (butter) beans, sorghum, cassava and linseed meal contain cyanide bound as glucosides. Rapeseed meal presents another problem due to the presence of glucosinolate. The enzyme myrosinase hydrolyses this to toxic isothiocyanates, oxazolidinethionines or nitriles and heat destruction of the enzyme reduces the toxicity [430].

TABLE 2.1. Effect of heat on the quality of legume proteins
(Hellendoorn *et al.*, 1971 [560])

	NPU	BV	Digestibility
Dun peas			
Raw	52	77	68
Boiled 5 min	55	82	67
Boiled 10 min	50	80	63
Heated 120°C for 120 min	37	75	49
White beans (Michigan pea bean)			
Raw	15	37	41
Boiled 5 min	48	71	68
Boiled 10 min	53	80	66
Boiled 60 min	49	77	64
Heated 120°C for 120 min	38	76	50

When these toxins are themselves proteins they are inactivated by heat; in other instances they may also be heat sensitive or they may have to be removed during processing.

The effects of heating legumes is illustrated by the figures in Table 2.1 [560]. The nutritive value of white beans (Michigan pea bean) was improved by 10 min boiling, whereas the Dun pea (*Pisum arvense*) was little affected. The improvement is due to destruction of toxins, including a haemagglutinin. The fall in nutritive value by heating at 120°C was due to reduced digestibility and there was no change in the biological value of the protein. Similarly, severe heat reduced the digestibility of the Dun pea with a possible small reduction in BV.

An example of the type of change involved is given by Anantharaman and Carpenter (1969) [397] using groundnuts. When fed to rats in the raw state they caused hypertrophy of the pancreas because of the trypsin inhibitor. Autoclaving or dry heat at 121°C for 30 min reduced the content of inhibitor to half but there was only a slight increase in nutritional value. When heating was continued for 4 hours there was a fall in available lysine with no change in methionine.

Neucere et al. (1972) [450] showed that there was no correlation between the amounts of trypsin inhibitor remaining after various heat treatments and the protein efficiency ratio.

Other foods

The beneficial effects of heat on foods other than legumes is not so well documented. Laporte and Trémolières (1962) [265a] reported the presence of a trypsin inhibitor in raw cereals such as rice, oats, maize, barley, wheat, rye and buckwheat. Cooking for 4 min at 98°C destroyed the inhibitor in wheat, rice and oats but not in the other grains. Hutchinson et al. (1964) [255] showed that barley is not improved by steaming and since barley does not form a gluten these authors suggested that the most likely explanation of the improvement of wheat on heating was increased digestibility resulting from the destruction of its capacity to form gluten. Cereals, in any case, are rarely eaten uncooked.

Hepburn et al. (1966) [252] reported changes in the availability of several amino acids on milling and baking of wheat. Methionine, tryptophan and threonine were more available in bread than in unground wheat; the availability of isoleucine incréased from 75% to 91% on milling and decreased to 70% on baking. The availability of leucine decreased from 94% to 75% on milling and increased to 100% on baking.

Another example of the beneficial effects of heat treatment is the inactivation of the mucoprotein, avidin, present in raw egg white. This can combine with the vitamin, biotin, and render it unavailable. Similarly some types of fish contain thiaminase which can destroy thiamin if the fish is eaten raw.

Niacin

Niacin is present in many cereals in a bound form which is not biologically available but can be liberated by heat, such as during baking, and under alkaline conditions. The classical example of the latter is the traditional process practised in Mexico of soaking maize in lime water before making tortillas.

The chemistry of this process explained a long-standing nutritional puzzle. It was known for many years that communities subsisting largely on maize as the staple food almost invariably suffered from pellagra. The niacin that is present is in a bound form and, at the same time, maize contains relatively little tryptophan, which can be converted into the vitamin. Yet pellagra was rare in Mexico, despite the widespread consumption of maize. The reason was that soaking in alkaline solution liberated the niacin.

As discussed in chapter 3 niacin is liberated when wheat flour is baked, especially with alkaline baking powder.

An additional and little recognised effect of processing is the formation of niacin in roasting of coffee. Darker coffees that have been more severely roasted are higher in niacin content because more of the trigonelline in the bean is converted into niacin.

Sprouting of seeds

It is common practice in many Eastern countries to sprout pea and bean seeds before consumption which leads to a marked increase in the vitamin C. Fordham *et àl.* (1975) [335] examined this procedure for a number of nutrients but the results are not directly comparable since, although the figures are calculated on a wet weight basis, the sprouted materials on average contain 90% water compared with an average of 6–10% for the seeds.

However, on the wet weight basis (which is the way in which the food is consumed) vitamin C increased up to ten-fold, thiamin fell to a quarter, tocopherol and niacin gave variable results in that some varieties of peas and beans showed an increase, some a decrease and some were unchanged. Riboflavin was unchanged.

Other beneficial effects

A minor example of a nutritional gain from food processing is the addition of trace minerals, such as calcium, from the processing water. Similarly the calcium content of meat is increased in methods of preparation that aid solution of calcium from the bone. Thus pork spareribs and chicken cooked with vinegar contain more calcium than the original muscle [104].

The use of vitamins C and E as processing aids can make a contribution to nutritional intake.

Phytate present in cereal bran and in mature legumes can reduce the absorption of iron, calcium and phosphate by forming insoluble salts, although the nutritional importance of this is not clear. However, phytate content can be reduced during processing.

Fermentation of cereals and pulses and various mixtures of the two, a traditional method of food processing in the East, can cause considerable increases in the amounts of riboflavin, niacin and vitamin B_6 (see p. 115).

There appears to be increased feed conversion efficiency when cereal feeding grains are heated [661]. The effect is believed to be due to the destruction of lipoxygenase, esterase and peroxidase which both confers greater stability on the product during storage and improves its palatability. Digestibility is not affected.

Section B

Effects on Nutrients

Chapter 3

VITAMINS

The vitamin content of raw foodstuffs can vary enormously – that of crops varies with variety, climate, soil, fertiliser, growing conditions and degree of maturity, that of animal foods varies with strain, age, nutrition and conditions of husbandry – so it is difficult to draw reliable conclusions from the mass of data available. Furthermore, post-harvest conditions and the methods of application of any specific process to the food vary so that the vitamin content of the end-product will cover a very wide range indeed.

The manufacturer requires to know both the extent of destruction during processing and the rate of loss during storage, particularly if he is making any claims for vitamin content, and so attempts have been made to study the kinetics of nutrient losses [540]. Data are very limited but some authors have produced mathematical models; for example nomographs have been produced for the losses of thiamin and ascorbic acid in canned foods but as discussed later [556, 735] they are not always applicable. It is often more useful to consider the properties of the individual vitamins as a guide to their stability in different foods under various conditions (Fig. 3.1).

Vitamin A

Vitamin A occurs in animal foods as retinol and in plant foods as a variety of carotenoids, chiefly β-carotene. It is added to many foods such as margarine, protein-rich baby foods, baking mixes, and, in special circumstances, to tea and to sugar.

The chemical structure of both carotenoids and retinol includes a series of conjugated double bonds so they are highly susceptible to oxidation. The purified and synthetic compounds are extremely unstable but in foods they are present in solution in the fats together with natural antioxidants and are more stable. Their oxidation depends on the rate of oxidation of the fats themselves since they are attacked by peroxides and free radicals formed from fats. Destruction, therefore, depends on temperature and access of air, and is promoted by light, traces of iron and especially traces of copper. Antioxidants that protect fats will also protect retinol and carotene.

Not being water-soluble there is no extraction of either form of vitamin A

27

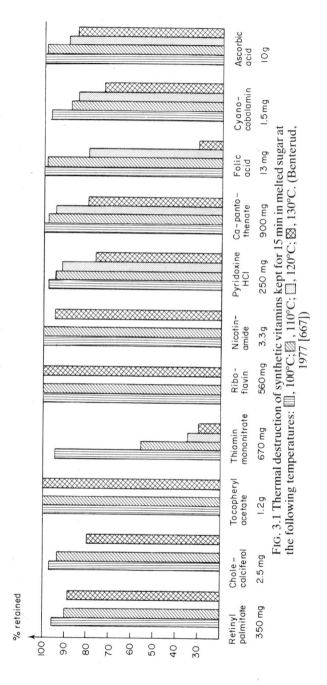

FIG. 3.1 Thermal destruction of synthetic vitamins kept for 15 min in melted sugar at the following temperatures: ▦, 100°C; ▨, 110°C; ▢, 120°C; ▧, 130°C. (Benterud, 1977 [667])

in wet-processing. Both are stable to pH changes except that there is some degree of isomerisation from all-*trans* to the less potent *cis*-forms at pH 4.5 or less [669].

In Western diets about one-third of the vitamin is present as retinol and two-thirds as carotene; in developing countries the greater part or even all the vitamin is supplied by plant foods. An example of western countries is Great Britain where 25% of the average intake comes from liver, 20% from butter and enriched margarine and 10% from milk; one single food, carrots, is so rich a source that it supplies 15% of the total intake.

TABLE 3.1. Loss of retinol (data compiled by De Ritter, 1976 [669])

	Storage (°C)	Loss (%)
Butter	1 year, 5	0–30
	5 months, 28	35
Margarine	6 months, 5	0–10
	6 months, 23	0–20
Skim milk powder	3 months, 37	0–5
	12 months, 23	10–30
Fortified cereal	6 months, 23	20
Fortified potato chips (crisps)	2 months, 23	0

TABLE 3.2. Loss of carotene (data compiled by De Ritter, 1976 [669])

	Storage (°C)	Loss (%)
Margarine	6 months, 5	0
	6 months, 23	10
Fortified lard	6 months, 5	0
	6 months, 23	0
Dried egg yolk	3 months, 37	5
	12 months, 23	20
Carbonated beverage	2 months, 30	5
Canned juices	12 months, 23	0–15

The stability of the vitamin varies with the food (see Tables 3.1, 3.2). It is very stable, for example, in liver; braised liver with internal temperature of 76°C lost 0–10% [47]. β-Carotene added to margarine at 500 ppm lost 40% during processing and a further 20% during 6 months storage at −20°C. Losses were the same from open packages and those sealed *in vacuo* [688]. Vitamin A appears to be very stable in butter – there was only 5% loss after 9 months at −18°C.

Boiling in water destroyed 16% of the vitamin A in margarine in 30 min, 40% in 1 hour and 70% in 2 hours. Frying at 200°C destroyed 40% of the vitamin A in enriched ghee and vanaspati in 5 min, 60% in 10 min and 70% in 15 min [687] see also Fig. 3.2.

Bector and Naranyanan (1975) [681] examined ghee prepared from both cow and buffalo milk for losses of carotene, retinol and vitamin E. Considerable destruction occurs when heated for 15 min at 150°C – 40% carotene, 30% retinol and 15% vitamin E in cow ghee and similar figures (there is no carotene present) in buffalo ghee. Carotene and retinol were

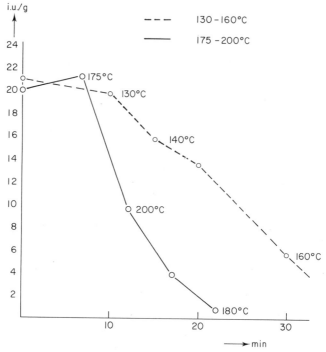

FIG. 3.2 Losses of vitamin A in margarine heated in a frying pan. (Benterud, 1977 [667])

completely destroyed in 15 min at 200°C or 60 min at 150°C, with 60% loss of vitamin E.

Milk suffers a loss of vitamin A on exposure to light – 10% was lost after 6 hours in sunlight [690a].

There is a slow loss of vitamin A added to powdered foods in the dry form. For example at 37°C after 9 months there was 25% loss of vitamin A, as well as 15% loss thiamin and 30% vitamin C [459, 889] but, as described below, stabilised forms are available.

The only major process that affects vitamin A is the drying and canning of fruits and vegetables.

Earlier results on losses of carotenoids are not valid for two reasons. In the older methods there were losses of carotene from enzymic degradation because the foods were not blanched. Secondly, the different carotenoids vary considerably in their biological potency and only total carotenoids were measured. The total was often unaltered, leading to the assumption that there had been no loss, but isomerisation into less potent forms of the vitamin does occur and was not realised in the earlier work [383].

Relative potencies of carotenoid isomers:

all-*trans* β-carotene	100
neo-β-carotene-B	53
all-*trans*-α-carotene	53
neo-β-carotene-U	38
neo-α-carotene-B	16
neo-α-carotene-U	13

The bulk of the carotenoids in fresh vegetables consists of the all-*trans* isomers and heat, such as during canning, converts part of these into neo-isomers with lower potency (e.g. all-*trans*-β-carotene into neo-β-carotene-U with only 38% activity) although as previously stated there may be no change in total carotenoid content.

Sweeney and Marsh (1971) [383] reported that processing reduced the vitamin A potency through isomerisation by 15–20% in green vegetables (containing mainly β-carotene) and by 30–35% in yellow vegetables (mainly α-carotene). Longer heating times increase the loss. The principal stereo-isomer in processed green vegetables is neo-β-carotene-U and in yellow and red vegetables is neo-α-carotene-B or neo-β-carotene-B. This work was carried out on a range of vegetables – broccoli, sprouts, spinach, collards, kale, beet greens, endive, carrots, squash, red peppers and pumpkin – which had been frozen or canned and subsequently cooked.

The same authors report that blanching and freezing of carrots and green vegetables does not cause any loss of potency.

Although higher temperatures and longer cooking times increase the losses of carotene there was found to be little practical difference between commercial canning and pressure cooking and conventional cooking. Since processed vegetables are already cooked this loss is an example of a processing loss that replaces domestic cooking loss and is not additional (depending on how much further heating the food suffers in the home).

Air-drying of vegetables and fruits can cause considerable losses, ranging from almost complete destruction in the old-fashioned open-air drying to 10–20% loss under controlled vacuum conditions. Pazarincevic-Trajkovic and Baras (1971) [373] found that carrots lost 40–50% of all their all-*trans*-β-carotene when dried in air, 20% when vacuum dried and 7% when dried in vacuum flushed out with nitrogen. The oxidation of vitamin A is promoted by heat and light.

During storage of dehydrated carrots there is a breakdown of carotene giving rise to an unpleasant flavour [333]: this can happen in a few days with powdered dehydrated carrots when there is a strong odour of violets presumably from the β-ionone formed (Bender, unpublished).

In general vitamin A is fairly stable under most conditions.

Stabilised and water-dispersible forms

Both retinol and carotene can be prepared as free-flowing powders that are stable to prolonged storage and are water dispersible, so can be added to aqueous foods. Retinol, as the acetate, and many of the carotenoids, are prepared in a starch-coated matrix of gelatin and sucrose together with added antioxidant [312]. The retinol can be used to enrich baby foods and similar mixtures and there is almost complete stability for periods up to one year at room temperature. It is also added to baking mixtures; there is a loss of 5–25% in baking.

The carotenes are used largely as colouring materials, rather than as sources of the vitamin, particularly to standardise the colour of fruit juices that may vary with season or source of supply. In such enriched fruit juices and concentrates the carotene is very stable, losses ranging from zero to 10% after one year's storage at 24°C.

Thiamin (Vitamin B₁)

Second only to vitamin C, thiamin is the most labile of the vitamins, being unstable at neutral and alkaline pH, catalysed by metallic ions such as copper. Since it is water-soluble it can be leached out of foods and this is probably the greater source of loss from most processed foods. It is stable to light and to acid, even at temperatures up to 120°C.

Dwivedi and Arnold (1973a) [695] reviewed the chemistry of its breakdown and Mulley *et al.* (1975) [707] reviewed the kinetics of the reaction.

It occurs in foods in three forms, as free thiamin, bound to pyrophosphate as cocarboxylase, and bound to protein, each with different degrees of stability. Mulley *et al.* (1975) [707] showed that the vitamin was more stable in food than in model buffer solutions which they attributed to the protection afforded by amino acids and proteins, and by adsorption on starch. The addition of proteins, gums and dextrins has some protective effect and the addition of cereals to pork has been shown to have a stabilising influence [81, 82].

A factor of considerable importance is that thiamin is completely destroyed by sulphur dioxide, since this is often used as a food preservative. It is also rapidly destroyed by oxidation by potassium bromate used as a bread improver but air itself usually has no important effect except, possibly, in dehydrated foods [698].

Some plant foods contain the enzymes thiaminase and polyphenolic oxidases which can destroy the vitamin; carrots, for example, have been shown to lose 50% of their thiamin in 90 days cold storage, while nearly all was lost from spinach kept 'in the shade' for 37 hours [564]. Enzymic destruction can be prevented by heat treatment.

1. *Solubility.* The main loss of thiamin from foods is by leaching into the processing and cooking water, depending, obviously, on the surface area. Chopped and minced foods can lose between 20 and 70% of their thiamin but this is recovered if the extracted liquor is consumed.

Some of the major dietary sources of thiamin such as cereals, do not undergo wet processing; other foods, for example pulses, present only a small surface area and little is extracted.

One of the most important sources of thiamin is meat and losses occur partly through heat destruction but mainly by loss of water-soluble extractives in the exuded juices. The most extreme example is, perhaps, the manufacture of meat extract. Here the meat is chopped into small pieces (0.5–1 cm cubes) and boiled for periods up to 15 min, when 80% of the water-soluble vitamins and muscle extractives can be removed.

A great deal of work has been carried out on the extrusion of meat juices during cooking – pan drippings. The amount is much greater at 200°C than at 105°C; since the principal factor is the internal temperature much will depend on the size of the sample rather than merely oven temperature. Since meat juices are usually consumed vitamins in pan drippings are not lost but about 20% of the thiamin can be oxidised at 200°C.

Vegetables, which (except for potatoes) are not major sources of thiamin, lose considerable quantities of water-soluble nutrients during the blanching process that precedes drying and freezing. Clearly, minced, chopped or sliced foods will lose more but there are considerable losses even in foods with small surface area-to-volume ratio, e.g. losses of 20–30% from potatoes and carrots [545, 387]. Sliced ham has a relatively large surface area and losses reached 50% when slices were soaked for 4 hours, changing the water every hour [87].

2. pH. The effect of alkalinity is demonstrated by the destruction of thiamin during cooking of rice. Roy and Rao (1963) [285] found no loss when rice was boiled in distilled water, 8–10% loss in tap water and up to 36% loss in well water – so demonstrating that the loss was not by leaching. When large volumes of water were used as in preparing rice gruel, a common practice in India, the loss was 5% in distilled water and 80% in well water.

Destruction of thiamin during baking of wheat products can be considerable if alkaline baking powders are used; normally 15–25% is destroyed in baking, mainly in the crust, but this can rise to 50% under alkaline conditions [698].

3. *Sulphur dioxide.* Sulphite is commonly used as a preservative in comminuted meats and processed fruits and vegetables. Sulphur dioxide slowly destroys thiamin at pH 3, very rapidly at pH 5, and immediately at pH 6. Hermus (1970) [702] treated minced meat with 0.1% SO_2 and even at 4°C 90% was destroyed in 48 hours; most of the loss took place in the first hour. Even at concentrations as low as 0.04% SO_2, 55% of the vitamin was destroyed, and subsequent frying increased this figure to 90%.

Twenty-five per cent of the thiamin was lost from cabbage during blanching and dehydration and this loss was increased to 85% when sulphite was added to the blanching water [359, 372] (see also Potatoes, p. 161).

Food composition tables can provide misleading thiamin values for prepared foods if the figures are derived from the composition of the raw materials. For example, comminuted meat products are often preserved with sulphite in Great Britain but not in some other countries so the thiamin content of such products cannot either be calculated from the meat content nor taken from food tables compiled from analyses of untreated products.

4. *Heat and oxygen.* Baking of bread results in losses of 15–30%, mostly in the crust but after baking the thiamin is stable [306, 698]. Toasting destroys more of the vitamin – 10-30% was lost in one experiment in periods of 30–70 s [244]. Clearly destruction depends on the thickness of the slice, time, temperature and moisture content.

Cereals stored as whole grain can suffer a loss of thiamin depending on the moisture content. In one series of observations at 17% moisture (a high level) 30% was lost from wheat in 5 months; at the more usual moisture content of 12% the loss was 12%; and when the moisture was reduced to 6% there was no loss. It appears to be more stable in rice – no loss was observed for periods up to 2 years [220, 241]. Thiamin-fortified white flour is stable for 6 months or more at room temperature [240].

Fortification is usually carried out with the hydrochloride; reports of the stability of thiamin mononitrate differ and it would appear that it is more stable than hydrochloride only under certain conditions (pharmaceutical preparations, chick diets); no difference was found between the two salts under other conditions (buffer solutions, yeast extract solutions, processed cheese) [698, 703]. Others have shown losses of mononitrate in enriched foods to be half those of the hydrochloride.

Stabilised nutrients

Thiamin is available in stabilised forms. For example, thiamin dicetyl sulphate is insoluble in cold water. Foods such as cereal grains can be enriched by soaking in such solutions of thiamin and they retain the added vitamin during any washing procedure. Similarly benzoylthiamin and the naphthalene-2,6-disulphonic acid derivative are used (U.S. Patent, 3 623 886, 1971).

An alternative method described in the same patent is to gelatinise rice grains by steaming so that the added thiamin and also added lysine are protected from leaching by the gelatinised coating.

Sulphite is often added as a preservative but destroys thiamin. A method of overcoming this drawback in dried potato is reported in U.S. Patent 3 343 970 – the vitamins are added to the potato at a stage removed from that of the addition of the sulphite. Only 8% of the added thiamin was lost in the process.

Encapsulated vitamins were used for enrichment in U.S. Patent 3 833 739, 1974. After 30 weeks storage at room temperature thiamin, riboflavin and niacin were quite stable; there was 25% loss of added ascorbic acid.

Beneficial effects of processing

Substances that destroy thiamin occur naturally in plants, for example 3,4-dihydroxycinnamic acid in fern and in blueberries, and chlorogenic acid, pyrocatechins and dihydroxycinnamic acid in coffee have antithiamin activity. Phenol derivatives with orthohydroxy groups have marked antithiamin activity, those with meta hydroxy groups have medium activity and those with parahydroxy groups are inactive. Polyphenol oxidase catalyses the degradation of thiamin by various plant phenols. Chan and Hilker (1976) were able to measure the amount of deactivated thiamin by fluorimetry. They showed that the rate of degradation by catechol increases with increasing pH linearly from pH 7 to 7.5 and that the rate of inactivation is independent of polyphenol oxidase concentration [693a].

Thiaminases, enzymes that destroy thiamin by splitting at the methylene bridge, have been found in various fish and crustaceans. Degradation leads to the formation of biologically inactive pyrimidine and thiazole. The latter confers a flavour on the food, the type of flavour apparently depending on the degree of purity of the substance – being sweet, meaty or pungent [838]. Heat destruction of thiaminases and polyphenol oxidase is obviously one of the advantages of processing.

Haeme protein present in beef, pork and tuna modify or destroy thiamin (Porzio et al., 1973) [709]. The authors raise the problem of analyses of thiamin content (or biological availability) in foods; most is present as pyrophosphate or bound to protein in which form it does not react with haeme, but when the thiamin is liberated during the analytical procedure, it may combine and lead to errors in analysis.

Kinetics of destruction

The loss of thiamin and ascorbic acid from foods during storage at constant temperature has been shown to be a first order reaction (but this may not hold under all conditions). Freed et al. (1949) [556] derived a nomograph for the loss of these two vitamins by storing foods at 21°C, 32°C and 38°C. The foods in question were, apricots, green beans, spinach, Lima beans, tomato juice, orange juice and peas. The nomographs are shown in Figs 3.3 and 7.2, p. 105, and according to the authors, results of other workers reported in the literature fitted well despite laboratory and experimental differences.

Farrer (1950) [697] used the factors he obtained in a study of the losses of thiamin from processed cheese, and from the assessment of published results on canned foods and dehydrated pork as a basis of calculation and suggested that this allows comparison of work carried out in different laboratories as well as enabling losses to be predicted.

However, Mulley et al. (1975) [707] concluded that although the destruction of thiamin measured in buffer solutions is a first order reaction, there are many deviations from this in foods. They state that it is still controversial whether destruction is purely thermal or whether oxidation is also involved.

Riboflavin (Vitamin B_2)

This occurs mostly bound with phosphate as flavin mononucleotide and as flavin adenine dinucleotide: it occurs in the free form in milk.

The amounts supplied in western diets are, on average, not much greater than recommended daily intakes and riboflavin deficiency is one of the commonest nutritional deficiencies in developing countries. Any processing loss is therefore a matter of concern.

Being water-soluble it can be leached into the processing water under the conditions discussed elsewhere (p. 97) but it is stable to oxygen and acid.

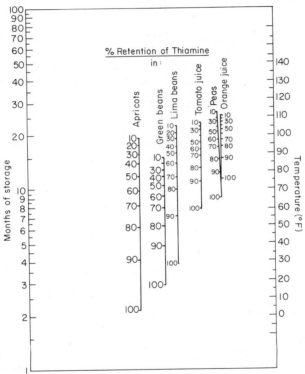

FIG. 3.3. Proposed nomograph for the stability of thiamin in canned foods. (Freed *et al.*, 1949 [556])

Heat alone does no damage even at 130°C but it is destroyed under alkaline conditions. In contrast with thiamin, sulphite has no effect [372].

Riboflavin is unusual in being sensitive to light and the food most affected is milk (as discussed on p. 133). In acid and neutral conditions light converts riboflavin to lumichrome; in alkaline solution to lumiflavin. The reactions are irreversible and temperature dependent; they appear to be first order reactions. Lumiflavin, in turn, destroys the vitamin C in milk and even small losses of riboflavin – about 5% – can lead to very large losses of vitamin C – 50%.

Light has also been shown to affect the riboflavin in small bread rolls. Three periods, each of 8 hours, exposure to light destroyed 17% of the riboflavin, reduced to 13% by wrapping in amber film and to 2% in orange film [293].

Niacin

Niacin occurs in foods in two forms, nicotinic acid and its amide, with the same biological activity; nicotinamide is usually present as the coenzymes, nicotinamide adenine dinucleotide (NAD) and its phosphate (NADP) but it is found in the free form in meat since the nucleotides break down after death of the animal.

In many cereals the vitamin is not biologically available since it is bound to polysaccharides and peptides, a combination originally termed niacytin [706]. The polysaccharide is cellulose or hemicellulose in type and is not hydrolysed during digestion. It is hydrolysed by acid and alkali, and Clegg (1963) [238] showed that 77% of the niacin of commercial wheat flour was unavailable but was liberated by baking with alkaline baking powder, the amount being dependent on time; it is completely liberated at pH 9.6.

In calculating the niacin content of a diet it is usual to ignore any cereals since, even after processing, it is not known how much might be available; free niacin added for enrichment is, of course, completely available.

The amino acid tryptophan can be converted into niacin in the body at the rate of 1 mg from 60 mg tryptophan so the vitamin content is usually expressed as niacin equivalents, which is the free vitamin plus 1/60th of the tryptophan.

Maize is poor both in free niacin and tryptophan and pellagra has long been common in areas where maize is the staple food. The Mexican practice of soaking maize in lime-water overnight before making tortillas liberates the vitamin and serves as a classic example of the benefits of food processing.

The amount liberated by heat varies with different foods; in roasted maize free niacin was increased thirty-fold, in Bengal gram by one-third and in rice by only one-tenth [711].

Consequently processing of cereal foods can give rise to extremely large losses of niacin during milling when the bran and germ are discarded, and an increase when heat or alkali treatment liberates the bound form.

So far as meat is concerned there is a loss of niacin (and the other B vitamins) into the expressed juices but so long as these are consumed together with the meat it is usually recovered. (See Meat, p. 123).

Niacin is very stable, the only losses in normal processing being by leaching into water. It is stable to heat, air and light at all pH's and is not affected by sulphite. Losses on blanching are similar to those of riboflavin – 10% from carrots, onions and potatoes, no loss from sweet potatoes [545]. In any case, vegetables are a poor source, cereals, especially the bran and germ, and meats being the most important sources.

Folic acid

Folic acid occurs in foods in a multiplicity of forms, differing in their biological potency and their stability. This is reflected in the variety of names that were given to this vitamin during its history (including vitamin B_c, factor M, Wills factor and *Lactobacillus casei* factor) and the still unresolved difference between the recommended nomenclature of the International Unions of Nutritional Sciences (IUNS) and Pure and Applied Chemistry (IUPAC).

	IUNS	IUPAC
Generic descriptor	Folacin	Folic acid
Specific compounds	Folic acid	Pteroylglutamic acid
	Folic acid (2)	Pteroyldiglutamic acid
	Folic acid (3)	Pteroyltriglutamic acid
	Tetrahydrofolic acid	Tetrahydropteroyl glutamic acid

The various forms are expressed as pteroylglutamic equivalents.

Folates occur in foods not only with varying numbers of glutamate residues but also as analogues with formyl, methyl and other groupings; 90% of the folate in cabbage is present in forms with more than 5 glutamate residues, 50% of that of soya contains monoglutamate, and in milk the conjugates range from mono- to heptaglutamates.

It is not clear whether these conjugates are biologically useful to human beings or whether only the free glutamate is available. According to the FAO/WHO Report of 1970 only the free form should be taken into account until more is known of the availability of the different forms and polyglutamates with more than three residues should be ignored. Human intestinal juice contains a conjugase which may liberate some part of the complex and some vegetables contain their own conjugases which may, when the food is macerated, liberate the free form of the vitamin, but the extent of this is not known.

The subject is further complicated by the absence of clear evidence of the daily requirements; the WHO Report of 1972 doubled the figures of the 1970 Report, apart from the problem of deciding which forms of the vitamin are available to man.

The assay of folate has been notoriously inaccurate for many years and, generally speaking, assays carried out prior to about 1970, when conditions were made more specific, are unreliable. For example, reports in 1950 gave the folate content of cow's milk at 1–2 μg per litre while those in the late 1960s gave values one hundred times as great [164], although the amount in milk is dependent to some extent on feed. Even apparently simple comparisons of the content of foods measured in the same laboratory before and after treatment can be in error since there might have been a differential breakdown of some of the conjugates of varying biological potency.

The vitamin is assayed microbiologically and problems arise from the response of different organisms to the various forms of the vitamin. *Streptococcus faecalis* does not respond to methyl folate, a form which is usable by man, but it does respond to pteroates which are not used by man. *Lactobacillus casei* assays appear to provide results closer to human utilisation.

This subject is a matter of considerable importance to food processors since it is believed (in view of the uncertainties listed above this word is used advisedly) that there is considerable loss during processing, and, at the same time, marginal deficiencies are thought to be widespread, at least among pregnant women, premature infants and possibly elderly people. Deficiency causes megaloblastic anaemia and sterility, and the newborn may suffer mental retardation. The richest sources are liver and kidney followed by dark green leaves: poorer sources are meat, fish, cereals and fruits.

Losses

Folate is relatively stable at slightly acid pH but unstable below pH 5, but the conjugates differ – monoglutamate is stable and tri- and hepta-glutamate are unstable to heat under acid conditions. Being water-soluble folate can be lost in wet processing and it is sensitive to heat. However, if cooking releases available vitamin from the larger polymers then there could be an increase in potency.

It can be destroyed by oxidation. For example the loss of folate from UHT milk during processing and subsequent storage depends on the amount of oxygen present and can vary between 20% and 100% (172).

It is protected by ascorbic acid which is added for this purpose to the assay medium. A similar protection appears to occur in foods since when milk is heated once, as in concentrating or drying, there may be no loss of folate, but subsequent reheating (e.g. in the preparation of infant formula) leads to progressive destruction. This is due to loss of the protective ascorbic acid in the first heating process [173].

Folate can also be destroyed by sunlight especially in the presence of riboflavin – one comparison showed a 30% loss in one year in tomato juice stored in clear glass bottles compared with only 7% in dark glass.

Hurdle *et al.* (1968) [720] reported no loss of folate on boiling or frying of chicken or liver, 90% loss on boiling or frying potatoes, 100% loss on boiling cabbage, 90% in spring greens, 70% on boiling and 30% on frying egg yolks.

An example of cumulative losses during processing was provided by Lin *et al.* (1975) [440]. Soaking of Garbanzo beans (*Cicer arietinum*) in water for 12 hours leached out 5%; blanching in water at 100°C caused a loss of 20% in 5 min, 25% in 10 min and 45% in 20 min. Sterilisation in the can at 118°C for 30 min destroyed a further 10%. Since folate is relatively stable at a slightly acid pH, such as existed in the can contents, a longer sterilising time did not lead to further loss.

Keagy *et al.* (1973) [259] found only 15% loss from wheat flour after 12 months storage at 29°C. At the much higher temperature of 49°C the loss

TABLE 3.3. Loss of folic acid (data collected by De Ritter, 1976 [669])

	Boiled (min)	Loss (%)
Cabbage	5	45
Potatoes	5	10
Liver	15	90
Meats	15	>50

was 40% after 1 month. Baking destroyed one-third of the folate naturally present but only 10% of the added folate. The latter was stable to storage in flour even at 50°C for 12 months and was not affected by potassium bromate, azodicarbonamide and benzoyl peroxide at the levels usually employed as bread improvers.

Losses from foods as diverse as vegetables, fruits and dairy produce average 70% of the free folate and 45% of the total folate during the overall processing and cooking stages. Malin (1975) [721] suggested that it is only the free folate that is labile and that combined forms are stable. He showed losses of 0–10% on steam blanching, 20% on pressure cooking and 25–50% on boiling – the amount lost being independent of the time of boiling. There were no losses during frozen storage and subsequent cooking but Hoppner *et al.* (1973) [584] reported 22% loss of free folate during the reheating of 30 convenience foods.

Vitamin B$_6$

Vitamin B$_6$ exists in three forms, pyridoxine (also termed pyridoxol), pyridoxal and pyridoxamine. The first two are the major forms in plant foods and the last two in animal foods. About two-thirds is present in combination, except for milk, where 90% is present in the free form.

The assay, which is microbiological, is not very precise since the test organisms vary in their response to the different forms of the vitamin, and these might change during processing. For example, pyridoxal is largely changed to the amine during sterilisation of milk. Moreover, problems in interpretation arise concerning the availability of the various forms of the vitamin to man. Possible processing losses are important since there is evidence that the average intake of the vitamin in western countries is somewhat borderline, particularly during pregnancy.

Stability

Pyridoxine itself is very stable to heat, none is lost during sterilisation, but the amine and aldehyde are more sensitive. However it is less stable in milk and there are considerable losses when milk is sterilised or dried, thought to be due to reaction with the -SH groups of the proteins [714].

During storage the amine can complex with -SH compounds leading to the formation, for example, of bis-4-pyridoxyl disulphide with only 12–23% of the activity of vitamin B_6 in rats. Other reactions can take place between vitamin B_6 and amino acids and proteins forming Schiff's base but these are vitamin B_6-active [152].

Temperatures employed in cooking do not destroy any of the three forms of the vitamin, and they are stable to acid and alkali and oxidation. The main loss is due to solubility in water. For example, Raab et al. (1973) found no loss from Lima beans during the sterilisation stage of canning, only during blanching – 20% in water blanching and 15% in steam blanching [456].

Tepley and Derse (1958) found that half of the frozen vegetables that they examined lost 20–40% of their vitamin B_6 after cooking – greater losses at this stage than with thiamin and riboflavin. Lushbough et al. (1959) reported that half the B_6 was lost from meat during cooking but this, clearly, will vary greatly with conditions [57].

Schroeder (1971) reviewed the data on losses during processing and summarised them as 40% loss from canned meat, 60–80% from canned vegetables, 40–60% from frozen vegetables, no loss in dairy products and on drying meat. These figures are based on the average figures for raw and processed foods, not on controlled trials [846].

See p. 134 for the effect of severe heat treatment on the vitamin B_6 content of milk.

Bunting (1965) found that 50% was lost into the cooking water but the vitamin was very stable during storage; only 5% was lost from enriched corn meal stored for one year at 38°C and 50% RH, and there was no loss on baking [226].

As with many other nutrients there is considerable loss in the milling of white flour (Tables 3.4 and 3.5).

TABLE 3.4. Vitamin B_6 content of wheat flours of different extraction rates ($\mu g/g$) (Clegg *et al.*, 1958)

Ext. rate	$\mu g/g$	Loss (%)
Manitoba 100%	4.5	
85	1.95	57
80	1.2	74
70	0.73	16

TABLE 3.5. Loss of vitamin B_6 (data collected by De Ritter, 1976 [669])

	Treatment	Loss (%)
Enriched bread	Baking	0
Enriched maize meal	12 months 38°C	5–10
Enriched macaroni	12 months 38°C	0
Infant milk (formula)	Heat processed	50
Infant milk (dry)	Spray dried	20–30
Chicken	Canned	40
Chicken	Irradiated	30

Vitamin C

The loss of vitamin C from foods by cooking was described as long ago as 1920, many years before it had been isolated and even before there was a chemical method of assay by Chick and Dalyell (1920) [321]. These authors observed that despite a good supply of vegetables 40 out of 64 children in a hospital in Vienna developed scurvy and that the antiscorbutic activity of cabbage (measured biologically) was reduced by 70% when it was cooked for 20 min at 100°C, and by 90% when cooked for 60 min at 70–80°C. Since there was a second reheating process (not unknown in present-day catering practice) it is possible that all the vitamin had been lost by the time the food was eaten. It is evident from many reports during the following half century that this lesson has still not been learned.

The term vitamin C designates both ascorbic acid (AA) and dehydro-ascorbic acid (DHA). The former is readily and reversibly oxidised to the latter but DHA is heat labile and converted irreversibly into diketogulonic acid, which has no biological activity (Fig. 3.4). The thermal half-life of DHA at pH 6 is less than 1 min at 100°C, and 2 min at 70°C irrespective of the presence of oxygen.

Vitamin C is easily leached into processing water and, apart from that, it is by far the most labile of the vitamins. It can be destroyed within plant tissues by oxidising enzymes – ascorbic acid oxidase, peroxidase, cytochrome oxidase and phenolase – by non-enzymic browning [795] and by degradation to furfural in the absence of air [736]. It is oxidised by air, powerfully catalysed by copper and also by iron; it is not affected by light except in the presence of riboflavin when the destruction can be very rapid – a problem virtually limited to milk (see p. 134); it is relatively stable to ionising radiation.

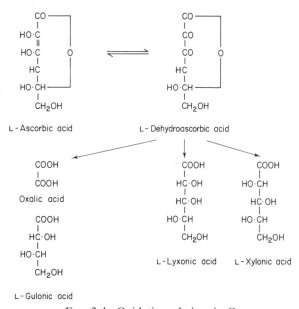

FIG. 3.4. Oxidation of vitamin C

Sulphite, often used in fruit juices as a preservative, protects vitamin C from oxidation. Dehydrated cabbage, for example, was shown to retain twice as much vitamin C when sulphited [372], although different authors report varying degrees of protection, possibly due to differences between foods as well as experimental conditions.

Assay methods

Figures for processing losses must take into account the method of assay used. There are three main methods. Perhaps the commonest is the dye-reduction of 2,6-dichlorophenolindophenol. This measures only the reduced form of ascorbic acid (and so may underestimate the total vitamin C activity) but also reacts with other reducing substances such as ferrous ions, reductones and sulphur dioxide (so may overestimate the vitamin).

The estimation with 2,4-dinitrophenylhydrazine requires the prior reduction of DHA to AA and so estimates both forms but can overestimate the potency by reacting with interfering substances – some of which are formed during heating and storage of foods. The most accurate method is by fluorimetry.

The errors involved in the older methods depend on the food in question. Clegg (1974) [577] reported that while the DHA content of vegetables is generally accepted as 2–3% of the total ascorbic acid content, and this was the value found in peas (and also by Somogyi *et al.* (1971) [494], in potatoes), it was 20% in green beans and 15% in Brussels sprouts. Hence the indophenol method might be applicable to some fresh vegetables but errors would arise in processed foods if some of the AA had been converted into DHA.

Enzymic destruction

Considerable amounts of vitamin C can be lost from fruits and vegetables during storage even before reaching the food processor. Bruising and wilting during transport and handling allow the oxidising enzymes access to the substrate and destroy the vitamin. It is also suggested that there are reductase systems which control the level of ascorbic acid. These are damaged when the fruit is bruised so that the oxidising enzymes can react with the ascorbic acid.

Ascorbic acid oxidase has its maximum activity at 40°C and is almost completely inactivated at 65°C, so rapid heating serves to protect the vitamin. This is the reason for blanching fruits and vegetables before drying or freezing (although there is a problem of possible regeneration of heat-inactivated peroxidases).

Birch *et al.* (1974) [315] pointed out that two reactions appear to be occurring simultaneously during heating – namely breakdown of the cell structure allowing contact between enzyme and substrate, and destruction of the enzyme. They found that in peas the point of maximum cell disruption and minimum rate of enzyme inactivation, i.e. fastest rate of oxidation of the vitamin, was 50°C. Leaching losses are also rapid when the cells are disrupted.

Enzymic destruction starts as soon as the crop is taken from the ground. For example, kale can lose 1.5% of its vitamin C per hour – about one-third in 24 hours. Losses are reduced by factors that reduce wilting such as high humidity and cool storage conditions. Green beans stored for only 24 hours at room temperature lost 24% of their vitamin C; this was reduced to 10% at 10°C. Broccoli lost 50% in 24 hours and 80% in 96 hours; the losses were reduced to 10–30% and 25–40% respectively at 10°C [664]. Freezing, however, may burst cells and bring the enzyme into contact with the vitamin. Leafy vegetables cannot be stored at temperatures below freezing point without causing damage to the tissue and figures from Finland illustrate this [382]. At harvest Brussels sprouts contained 99–198 mg vitamin C per 100 g; after 60 days storage in open boxes at 1°C the content was 116 mg. It was the same if the temperature was maintained at −1°C for the 60 day period, but at −2.5°C the figure fell to 84 mg, and at −5°C to 31 mg.

Leaching losses

The blanching process necessary to destroy the oxidising enzymes causes considerable losses of vitamin C and other soluble nutrients by leaching [513] although alternative methods have been investigated in order to reduce these losses (Table 7.1, p. 99). The amount lost depends, among other factors, on the volume of water and the state of subdivision of the food rather than the time of treatment. For example, in one experiment vegetables covered with water lost 80% of their vitamin C; half-covered in water they lost 60%; quarter-covered, 40%. The amount of vitamin destroyed may be quite small compared with the amount leached out. In 10 vol. water a sample of cabbage lost 10% of the ascorbic acid by destruction and 80% into the cooking water. This is the basis of the domestic scientists' advice to make use of the water in which vegetables have been cooked. The commercial equivalent is the liquor in canned fruits and vegetables which may contain more vitamin C than the solids. Summary of findings are shown in Table 8.13, p. 152.

Oxidation

The marked effects of oxygen are shown by the virtual absence of vitamin C from sun-dried fruits and vegetables [365]. Vitamin C can be extremely stable when protected from air in cans or bottles and kept cool, and fruit juices are often additionally protected with sulphur dioxide. There may be loss immediately after canning or bottling due to dissolved and headspace air. Residual oxygen is normally used up in the electrochemical process of corrosion and so disappears rapidly in plain cans and much more slowly in lacquered ones and glass bottles. In consequence there is a greater loss of vitamin C in lacquered cans than in plain ones [309]. After the residual oxygen has been removed the vitamin C is usually stable for periods of several months.

Kefford *et al.* (1959) [353] found that pasteurised fruit juices lost vitamin C by oxidation during the first few days storage at 30°C, but after the oxygen had been used up there was an anaerobic loss proceeding at about one-tenth of this rate. Since the latter continued for a long period of time the anaerobic loss finally exceeded the aerobic loss.

In some processes the food is de-aerated. For example, orange juice extracted with a high-speed reamer is often supersaturated with air to 0.5% by volume; this can be reduced to 0.05% by de-aeration.

Anaerobic destruction is accelerated by sucrose, fructose and fructose phosphates leading to the formation of furfural [353]. This reaction is largely independent of pH but slightly increased in the range pH 3–4.

It is common practice in the United States to add sufficient vitamin C to allow for a loss of 8–15 mg per 100 g fruit juice in processing and 12 months storage; this is an absolute amount irrespective of initial concentration of the

TABLE 3.6. Percentage loss of vitamin C from fruit squash exposed to air (Bender, 1958 [313])

	8 days	15 days	35 days	40 days
Stored full	5		10	
Opened	15	30		90
Stored half full	30	60	70	100

vitamin. Fruits rich in anthocyanins appear to lose vitamin C more rapidly – strawberries can lose 40–60% on processing and 4 months storage at 37°C [341]; raspberries and blackcurrants are even less stable. Some fruit preparations have been found to be very unstable; Noel and Robberstad (1963) [368] found that orange juice stored at 5°C lost 3–30% of the vitamin C in 16 days, and that apple juice lost 50% in 4–8 days and 95% in 16 days.

The variation between samples stored under the same conditions suggests that there are other factors involved. Bender (1958) [313] found a two-fold range in vitamin C content of a fruit squash preparation within a batch of experimental samples stored under identical conditions, and drew attention to a similar finding within bottled fruits. Harris and Von Loesecke (1960) [895] make the same point when they state that published data suggest that the influence of temperature on thiamin stability may vary from pack to pack of a specified canned food.

While the vitamin C may be very stable during storage in a sealed container, especially if sulphur dioxide is present, there is a very rapid destruction as soon as the container is opened and the vitamin comes into contact with air [313]. Table 3.6 shows that 30–50% of the vitamin C can be lost within 8 days and as much as 90% after 3–4 weeks.

Kinetics of destruction reactions

The rates of destruction of vitamin C have been shown by some authors to follow a first order reaction but there appear to be different mechanisms operating in different foods. Freed *et al.* (1949) [556] produced a nomograph for the rates of destruction of ascorbic acid under a variety of conditions (Fig. 7.2), and Wanninger (1972) [735] also produced a mathematical model taking account of temperature, water and oxygen, using the reported values of Vojnovich and Pfeifer (1970) [302] as evidence to support his equations.

However, Labuza (1972) [539] pointed out that there are several anomalies in the published reports of vitamin C destruction which could be explained by different mechanisms. In addition to oxidation, losses of ascorbic acid in some foods run parallel to the extent of non-enzymic browning. In this reaction the activation energy increases with decreasing moisture while the loss from enriched wheat flour and a corn-soy-milk mixture decreased with decreasing moisture. In orange juice crystals losses were the same in air and in vacuum and there were losses even below the monolayer of moisture. Labuza suggests that the mechanism of ascorbic acid destruction may differ at different moisture contents – possibly oxidation being the main cause of destruction at low moisture and browning at high moisture content. The loss of added ascorbic acid from wheat flour and corn-soy-milk mixture and from cabbage was a first order reaction, and increased with temperature. The rate of loss from carrot flakes, however, was not affected by temperature [380].

The difficulty of producing a mathematical model in the present state of knowledge is illustrated by the observations of Marchesini *et al.* (1975) [442], (Table 1.6). They showed that even among a range of fifteen cultivars of green beans grown under identical conditions the rates of loss of both ascorbic and dehydroascorbic acid differed enormously. Under the same conditions (canning: 8 min at 124°C) one cultivar lost all the AA and three-quarters of the DHA, while another lost only one-quarter of the AA and a quarter of the DHA. At a lower temperature (25 min at 116°C) the latter cultivar lost more AA than the former cultivar but less DHA. Yet another difference is that the amount of vitamin leached into the brine in the cans differed among the cultivars.

Stable forms

The sulphate (L-ascorbate 2-sulphate) (used to avoid colour changes in grape juice) is much more stable than the free acid but its biological activity has not been established in man. It will withstand baking at 218°C for 15 min [731, 732]; the dipotassium L-ascorbate sulphate loses only 15% under these conditions compared with 65–90% loss of free ascorbic acid. The loss of the sulphate is independent of concentration because it is a zero-order reaction, while loss of the free acid decreases with increasing concentration since its destruction depends on the ascorbic acid oxidase present in the wheat flour. In pancakes the loss of the sulphate was only 5% whereas that of the free acid was 100%.

When added to milk and stored at 10°C, only 5% of the sulphate was lost compared with 30% of the free acid.

Ascorbic acid beadlets protected with gelatin/starch are used to enrich foods like cereals and milk powder. Bauernfeind and Pinkert (1970) [724] showed that after 12 months storage at 23°C losses were 5–30% from a range of cereal, milk and fruit products.

TABLE 3.7. Stability of vitamin C in various carriers. Loss after 1 year storage in closed bottles (from Kläui, H. [727])

(Water content %)	Wheat starch (12)	Wheat flour (12.5)	Skim milk (3.5)	Glucose monohydrate (9)	Glucose anhydrous (0.1)
Ascorbic acid RT	2	30	30	25	3
45°C	16	30	30	25	25
Sodium ascorbate RT	2	30	20	25	5
45°C	20	30	28	25	25
Ascorbyl palmitate					
RT	4	30	14	10	14
45°C	15	60	20	45	20

Table 3.7 shows the marked effect of the carrier on the stability of added vitamin C [727]. Crystals coated with triglyceride or with ethocel have been shown to be stable.

Vitamin C as a processing aid

Quite apart from nutritional enrichment vitamin C is used as an antioxidant and a stabiliser in many foods and drinks, to improve the baking quality of flour and in curing meat products [561, 724, 727].

Fruits and beverages. The browning of fruits and fruit juices is caused by the enzyme polyphenoloxidase which converts orthophenols to ortho-quinones in the presence of oxygen. While it can be destroyed by heat this might produce unwanted flavours, or, in the case of fruits, spoil the texture: either sulphur dioxide or ascorbic acid can serve as an inhibitor. Sulphur dioxide is an enzyme inhibitor; the ascorbic acid functions by reducing the substrate after it has been oxidised by the enzyme. Relatively large quantities are needed of the order of 150–200 mg per litre. About two-thirds of this might still remain after processing and storage so this method of preservation results in a substantial nutritional contribution [727].

Similarly ascorbic acid is used in frozen and canned fruit, frozen fish (1 g/kg), for pickling olives in brine, sauerkraut and various vegetables. It is also used to some extent in preserved chipped potatoes that have been cooked and stored frozen. It serves to prevent browning of the potato and also acts as an antioxidant in the frying oil. It does not appear to be useful in preventing the browning of raw potatoes [727].

Ascorbic acid is used at concentrations of 20–40 mg/litre in the brewing of beer as an oxygen acceptor to prevent changes in flavour and colour and to reduce chill and oxidation haze. It is also added to wine at the rate of 50–100 mg/l to preserve taste and colour and to prevent ferric phosphate turbidity by reducing the salt to the more soluble ferrous form.

Meat products. The red colour of meat can be controlled by ascorbic acid functioning as a reducing agent. Meat is preserved by curing with salt, nitrate and nitrite – the nitrate/nitrite are essential for colour development. Nitrate is converted into nitrite by microorganisms which then react with muscle myoglobin to form the desired red nitrosomyoglobin. After cooking the colour remains when the compound is converted into nitro-somyohaemochrome.

This series of reaction is relatively slow and for quick curing it is necessary to provide a reducing agent – ascorbic acid reduces metmyoglobin to myglobin so that it reacts with nitric oxide; nitric oxide is formed from nitrite by ascorbic acid. Two additional advantages are that less nitrite is necessary and the colour is developed more evenly. Moreover, the addition of vitamin C is recommended as a method of blocking the formation of possibly carcinogenic nitrosamines from nitrite and amines. Since this reaction can possibly occur *in vivo* after eating cured meats, it is obviously essential that the ascorbic acid survives processing. Newmark *et al.* (1974) [68] fried bacon for 6 min at 170°C and found that 20–30% was destroyed; storage of bacon resulted in losses of 1% per week in the freezer and 8% per week in the refrigerator.

The amounts of ascorbic acid used are 150–500 mg per kg meat, depending on the colour required. At the end of the process and after storage there is still vitamin C left which may be of great nutritional benefit to those individuals who eat very little fruit and vegetables.

Flour and bread. Flour 'improvement' which enhances bread texture and loaf volume is caused by oxidation of sulphydryl compounds to disulphides (–SH to –S–S–) and this can be effected with ascorbic acid. (The first step is oxidation of the ascorbic acid to dehydro form which then functions as an oxidising agent.) The amounts are relatively small (10–50 ppm in bulk fermentation and 50–200 ppm in continuous bread process and 75 ppm in the Chorleywood process) and the vitamin is destroyed in baking so that it is not of any nutritional importance [298]. In a fat-soluble form such as the palmitate, ascorbic acid is effective as a fat antioxidant, particularly when used synergistically with α-tocopherol and gallates. The amounts used are about 500 ppm ascorbyl palmitate and 200 ppm tocopherol so that there may be a significant amount of vitamins available from such enriched fats, even after some loss through oxidation.

Conclusion

Since vitamin C is the most labile of the nutrients its loss is sometimes used as an index of damage to other nutrients. This is likely to be true only in that if there is little loss of vitamin C then it is reasonably certain that there is little or no loss of other nutrients, but it is not true that destruction of vitamin C indicates a loss of other nutrients – in many foods vitamin C is the only nutrient that is lost.

It must be concluded that much of the loss of vitamin C is inevitable in almost every type of food preparation and although it may be minimised by good manufacturing practice the losses must always be considerable. At the same time the widespread use of vitamin C as a processing aid will, to some extent, remedy this loss. In the instance of meat products there is a real nutritional benefit from the processing since there are a number of individuals who eat virtually no fruits and vegetables and who could obtain the greater part of their daily needs of vitamin C from such processed meats.

Vitamin D

This is generally regarded as being fairly stable but the difficulties of assay mean that little information is available. It is considered to be similar to vitamin A in being destroyed in oxidising fats but it has been shown to withstand the smoking of fish, pasteurisation and sterilisation of milk and spray drying of egg.

Vitamin D is often added to infant formulas and it has been common practice, based on a limited number of assays, to allow for the destruction of 25–35% of the vitamin during the drying process.

Vitamin E

The importance of vitamin E in the human diet has not been clearly established – dietary deficiencies never seem to occur even in developing countries. On the other hand it is a dietary essential and it has been shown that an increase in the amount of polyunsaturated fats in the diet increases the requirement of vitamin E.

There are eight compounds included in the vitamin E group (α-, β-, γ- and δ-tocopherols and α-, β-, γ- and δ-tocotrienols) each with a different biological potency. It is usual to express the vitamin E activity of foods in terms of α-tocopherol equivalents; the biological potency of α-tocopherol is therefore 1.0; that of γ-tocopherol is 0.08; α-tocotrienol is 0.21 and γ-tocotrienol is 0.01.

TABLE 3.8. Vitamin E content of fresh and canned vegetables (after Bunnell *et al.*, 1965 [740])

	Total tocopherol mg (%)	α-Tocopherol mg (%)
Fresh green peas	1.73	0.55
Canned green peas	0.04	0.02
Frozen green beans	0.24	0.09
Canned green beans	0.05	0.03
Frozen kernel corn	0.49	0.19
Canned kernel corn	0.09	0.05

Thus assay for vitamin E requires separate measurements of the different compounds and recoveries are of the order of only 55–65%. This means that small changes after processing may have no significance.

Being fat-soluble vitamin E is not lost by leaching in processing water and is generally stable. It is, of course, a naturally occurring anti-oxidant in many vegetable oils and therefore preferentially destroyed under oxidising conditions such as exposure to air and light, accelerated by heat and copper. However, such changes are relatively slow and processing damage is insignificant. For example, little is lost from vegetable oils even at frying temperatures. On the other hand there is a considerable loss from fried foods during frozen storage – conditions under which most other nutrients are stable. Bunnell *et al.* (1965) [740] showed that while the oil used for frying lost 10% of its vitamin E content in the process, the oil absorbed into the food lost vitamin E rapidly when stored at $-12°C$. Potato chips (crisps) lost 48% in two weeks at room temperature rising to 70% in 4 weeks and 77% in 8 weeks. Stored at $-12°C$ the loss was just as rapid (63% in 4 weeks and 68% in 8 weeks). Similarly French fried (chipped) potatoes lost 68% of the vitamin E (absorbed from the cooking oil) in 4 weeks and 74% in 8 weeks frozen storage.

This loss is believed to be caused by the formation from unsaturated fatty acids of hydroperoxides which are relatively stable at the low temperature. Normally they decompose to peroxides, then to aldehydes and ketones which are less damaging to the vitamin E.

Free tocopherol is slowly oxidised in air while the esters are more stable. For example, Bunnell *et al.* (1965) showed that tocopherol acetate was only 10–20% destroyed under conditions where free tocopherol was completely destroyed [740].

Boiling destroys 30% of the tocopherol in sprouts, cabbage, carrots and leeks [317] and the losses on canning are considerable (Table 3.8). However, vegetables are not an important source of vitamin E in the human diet.

Moore *et al.* (1957) reported 50% destruction during bread-making through the use of chlorine dioxide as a flour bleaching agent [743].

Other vitamins

A number of vitamins are of medical rather than nutritional interest since dietary deficiencies rarely arise. Consequently processing damage is probably of less importance and has been less intensively investigated. These include pantothenic acid, biotin, vitamin K, *p*-amino benzoic acid and cyanocobalamin.

Pantothenic acid exhibits optimal stability at pH 6–7 and is stable at higher pH but is more sensitive in acid media at pH 3–4. It is stable to oxygen and light but not to heat.

Morgan *et al.* (1944) [545] showed that there were no losses of pantothenate in blanching of carrots and potatoes, on drying potatoes, and only 5% loss from sweet corn and 10% from onions on drying. Other work on this vitamin is referred to under Effects of Processes and Commodities.

Cyanocobalamin (*vitamin B$_{12}$*) is generally heat stable at acid pH but there is a 10% loss from milk during 'holder' pasteurisation due to interaction with vitamin C and sulphydryl compounds from denatured protein and glutathione. As discussed under Milk (p. 136) this loss does not occur in the absence of oxygen.

It is affected by oxidising and reducing agents. Frozen meat and fish dishes can lose up to 20% of the vitamin. Being water-soluble it is extracted into the cooking water and meat juices can contain up to 30% of the cyanocobalamin of the meat – this is recovered if the juices are consumed.

Since it is stable to heat in neutral and acid media there is little loss in canning, generally about 10–20%.

TABLE 3.9. Percentage vitamin losses (from Thomas and Calloway, 1961 [547])

		Thiamin	Riboflavin	Niacin	Pyridoxine	Pantothenate	Folate	Tocopherol
Bacon								
Raw (amount present)		370 µg	132 µg	2.4 mg	—	400 µg	—	0.6 mg
Crisped at 176°C	(1)	5	(+70)*	(+60)*		(+80)*		(+10)*
Fried at 288°C	(2)	5	(+80)*	(+50)*				
Beef								
Raw (amount present)		52 µg	170 µg	4.1 mg	300 µg	460 µg	3 µg	0.8 mg
Boiled 55 min	(3)	30	0	10	10	25	0	50
Same freeze dried then reheated	(4)	90	0	50				
Canned and fried	(5)	80	0	10	40	20	10	65
Chicken								
Raw (frozen) (amount present)		57 µg	175 µg	6.9 mg	500 µg	960 µg	4 µg	0.4 mg
Simmered 50 min	(6)	50	30	40	95	50	20	30
Same freeze-dried rehydrated, boiled 30 min	(7)	55	70	60				
Boiled 35 min canned	(8)	98	15	20	30	30	0	50
Same reheated 30°, contents drained	(9)	98	(+10)	30				
Pork loin								
Raw (amount present)		870 µg	210 µg	4.8 mg	440 µg	700 µg	<1 µg	0.40 mg
Fried and canned	(10)	70	0	10	50	50	—	60
Same reheated	(11)	85	(+20)*	10	50			

Shrimp

	18 µg	19 µg	0.9 mg	80 µg	200 µg	3 µg
Raw (frozen) peeled (amount present)	18 µg	19 µg	0.9 mg	80 µg	200 µg	3 µg
Boiled 4 min (12)	50	0	60	20	80	50
Same rehydrated 15 min (13)	50	(+20)*	70	–	–	–
Boiled 10 min, canned (14)	80	0	80	60	0	60

Vitamin C

Carrots

Raw (amount present)		6 mg
Boiled 5 min, dried	(15)	30
Same cooked 12 min	(16)	70
Steamed 15 min, dried	(17)	20
Same boiled 20 min	(18)	70
Steamed 5 min, canned	(19)	50
Same reheated	(20)	80

Corn

Raw (frozen) amount present		9 mg
Vacuum-dried	(21)	35
Simmered 30 min	(22)	30
Steamed 12 min	(23)	40
Standing in hot water 25 min	(24)	65
Steamed and canned	(25)	40
Same reheated	(26)	60

Green beans

Fresh-frozen (amount present)		4 mg
Steamed 4 min, dried	(27)	70
Simmered 10 min	(28)	70
Steamed 9 min, freeze-dried	(29)	70
Same reconstituted	(30)	80
Steamed 4 min, canned	(31)	75
Same reheated	(32)	75

Cabbage

Raw (amount present)		42 mg
Dehydrated	(33)	10
Boiled 10 min	(34)	50
Steamed 3 min, dried	(35)	25
Same reheated	(36)	60

* See Processing methods (9).

Processing methods

Bacon
    (1)   Cooked 176°C in oven until crisp
    (2)   Broiled at 288°C 4 min one side, $1\frac{1}{2}$ min on the other
Beef
    (3)   Cooked at 100°C 55 min, internal temp 62–68°C
    (4)   As (3), subsequently sliced freeze-dried, then rehydrated 20 min and grilled at 232°C 2 min each side of slice
    (5) $3\frac{1}{4}$ oz patties fried in deep fat 1 min 20 s at 176°C, canned and cans heated at 121°C 90 min
Chicken
    (6)   Simmered 50 min, skinned and boned
    (7)   (6) freeze dried, subsequently rehydrated 30 min boiling salt solution
    (8)   Cooked in a retort on trays at 100°C 35 min, boned, canned and heated $2\frac{1}{2}$ h 115°C
    (9)*   (8) reheated 30 min boiling water; the high riboflavin content compared with 8 is explained by the authors as either due to the formation of fluorescent compounds or the release of a bound form of riboflavin
Pork loin
    (10)   Sliced $\frac{5}{8}$ inch thick, fried deep fat 176°C; canned, heated 121°C 50 min
    (11)   (10) reheated 30 min boiling water
Shrimp
    (12)   Cooked 4 min boiling water (freeze-dried)
    (13)   (12) rehydrated 15 min cold water
    (14)   Blanched in boiling brine 10 min, canned, heated 25 min 116°C
Carrots
    (15)   Sliced $\frac{1}{8}$–$\frac{3}{16}$ inch thick, steamed 100°C 5 min, dipped in sulphite solution 1 min, vacuum dried
    (16)   Dried product cooked by adding to cold water, boiling and simmering 12 min
    (17)   Steamed 100°C 15 min, vacuum dried
    (18)   Dried product cooked by boiling 20 min
    (19)   Steamed 5 min, canned 116°C 30 min
    (20)   Canned product reheated 82°C (time not stated) and drained
Corn
    (21)   Dipped in sulphite solution $1\frac{1}{2}$ min, vacuum dried
    (22)   Cooked by adding to boiling water, standing 30 min, simmering 20 min
    (23)   Steamed 12 min, sprayed with sulphite solution, freeze-dried
    (24)   Cooked by adding to boiling water and standing 25 min
    (25)   Steamed 4 min, canned 116°C 25 min
    (26)   Reheated at 82°C (time not stated) and drained
Green beans
    (27)   Steamed 4 min 100°C, dipped 2 min in sulphite solution freeze-dried
    (28)   Cooked by adding to boiling water and simmering 10 min
    (29)   Steamed 9 min and freeze-dried
    (30)   Reheated by adding to boiling water and standing 25 min
    (31)   Steamed 4 min, canned 116°C 25 min
    (32)   Reheated 82°C (time not stated) and drained

Cabbage
- (33) Dipped 1 min in sulphite solution, vacuum dried
- (34) Cooked by boiling 10 min
- (35) Dipped 1 min in sulphite solution, steamed 100°C 3 min, vacuum dried
- (36) Reheated by adding to boiling water and standing 10 min and draining

Cyanocobalamin can be destroyed in solution by vitamin C and the same effect appears to take place in foods containing the two vitamins [701]. The observation that large oral doses of vitamin C lowered the blood levels of vitamin B_{12} suggests that destruction can also take place *in vivo*.

Small amounts of iron stabilise B_{12}, larger amounts cause a loss; foods containing both iron and vitamin C may have unpredictable amounts of B_{12} left.

Biotin (*vitamin H*) is stable to heat, dilute acids and alkalis, oxygen and light but can be inactivated by lipid peroxides. Braekkan and Boge (1960) [111] found it stable in fish on canning and in milk on sterilising and drying.

Deficiencies of biotin occur in human beings only under bizarre conditions where raw egg white is consumed in large quantities. This is due to binding to the protein, avidin, and since this is denatured by heat and cannot then bind the biotin, heat processing is beneficial.

Chapter 4

PROTEINS

Two apparently contradictory conclusions can be drawn from the evidence in the literature, namely, that except in special circumstances most processes have little effect on protein quality and, on the other hand, proteins can readily be damaged even under mild conditions. One overall conclusion is that when damage does occur it is usually of little practical nutritional importance (so far as we know).

Most processes such as dehydration, canning and domestic cooking have, in general, only a small effect on protein quality but this is a generalisation to which there are many exceptions. Specialised processes involving high temperatures such as the puffing and roasting of cereals and the poorly controlled drying of animal feedstuffs such as fish meal and oil seed residues do cause damage.

Much of the work has been carried out on lysine and this has given rise to a general impression that lysine is the only amino acid to suffer damage. While under some conditions it is the most sensitive amino acid others are also affected, especially cystine and methionine. Those with reactive side chains such as epsilon amino, guanidyl, indole (i.e. lysine, arginine, tryptophan and histidine) can form linkages with reducing substances present in the food and are not liberated by the digestive enzymes i.e. they are 'biologically unavailable'.

Pieniazek *et al.* (1975) [816] reported a considerable reduction in availability of eleven amino acids when casein was heated with glucose for 24 h at 90°C in the presence of 4% moisture. The availability of methionine was reduced to 25%, aspartic acid, glutamic acid, threonine, serine, glycine, histidine and arginine to 25–30%, and lysine and alanine to 85% of the initial values. These losses were greatly increased at 80% moisture when there was a fall in the availability of all the amino acids except tyrosine and phenylalanine, and these were also affected when glucose was added.

Loss of *total* amino acid was very much less; at 4% moisture in the absence of glucose there was 10–20% destruction of cystine, methionine, tyrosine, lysine and arginine. The addition of glucose at this moisture content doubled the destruction of lysine (from 13% to 22%) but did not affect the losses of other amino acids.

Protein terminology

Since investigators have used a variety of methods of assessing the nutritional value of proteins a brief description of terminology may be helpful.

It must be emphasised that much of the discussion relating to the loss of quality of one single food is somewhat academic since it is the quality of the combined proteins of the whole diet (and also the protein–energy ratio) that is of interest. For example individual foods have qualities ranging from net protein utilisation (NPU) 1.0 to zero. Yet the overall quality of the diets of the western world is NPU 0.7–0.8, and that of the poorest diets of the world is 0.6, and only occasionally as low as 0.5.

In other words the supplementation of basic cereal (or even root crop) diets with such high quality proteins as meat and milk does not increase the NPU by more than about 20%. Conversely, damage to any one protein food would have only a small effect on the quality of the total diet. Moreover, in countries where processing is common the diet usually contains a relative surplus of protein so that loss of quality is not important, at least for adults.

Nevertheless, from the point of view of good manufacturing practice, not to mention marketing, it is necessary to ensure that food suffers as little damage as possible during processing, and there may well be sections of a community where reduction in protein quality is a hazard.

Available amino acids

In stored and heated proteins part of the amino acids may become linked to other substances by bonds that are resistant to hydrolysis by the digestive enzymes, although they are liberated by acid hydrolysis. The information required, therefore, is the amount of each amino acid that is biologically available. Chemical analysis which is preceded by acid hydrolysis gives only the total amino acid content.

Measurement of availability usually requires biological methods since chemical methods are applicable only to lysine and even in this instance there are exceptions (Carpenter and Booth, 1973).

Lysine has two amino groups, the alpha group linked with the adjacent carboxyl group of the next amino acid in the polypeptide chain, and the free epsilon-amino group projecting from the chain. It is when this epsilon-amino group becomes linked in a form that is resistant to the digestive enzymes that the lysine becomes unavailable.

Chemical methods of determining free epsilon amino groups reveal the amount of available lysine. The method largely in use [763] depends on their reaction with fluorodinitrobenzene (available lysine value–ALV). The method works well with animal sources of protein and is a valuable means of monitoring processing changes but unfortunately large amounts of carbohydrate interfere with the reaction so that it is not applicable to cereals:

Other chemical methods are also under investigation (Carpenter and Booth, 1973 [809]).

A simple method of following changes in overall reactive amino groups, including the side chains of arginine and histidine, is the uptake of dyes such as Orange G. Dye-binding is of value in following changes in particular foods but cannot be used with any reliability for comparing the nutritional value of different foods [800].

Amino acid pattern

In many lightly processed foods where the greater part of all the amino acids is available the amino acid pattern determined after hydrolysis is a useful index of nutritional quality. The amounts can be compared with recommended intakes. Such figures are, however, considered only as a guide and usually verified biologically.

Conversion factor

Since proteins differ in their amino acid composition and therefore in their nitrogen content the factor for converting chemically determined nitrogen into protein differs with the protein. It is 6.38 for milk, 5.3 for some legumes, 5.7 for cereals and 6.25 for many other food proteins. There is no general agreement on which factor should be used for mixtures although 6.25 is commonly used.

Consequently it is not quite correct to express the amino acids as a percentage of the protein, although this is often done. A common convention is to express each of them as g amino acid per 16 g total nitrogen – which is the same as per cent amino acid assuming a conversion factor of 6.25. Some authors quote figures as g amino N per g protein N, or mg amino acids per 100 g protein or per 100 g food.

Net protein utilisation – NPU

This is the proportion of the dietary protein that is retained in the body for all purposes (growth, repair, production of enzymes, etc.). Earlier publications express both net protein utilisation and biological value as percentages but with the S.I. system they are expressed as ratios i.e. NPU 50% is now expressed as 0.5. Since it is nitrogen that is measured the question of the conversion factor is not involved.

The method requires measurement either of the difference between nitrogen consumed and that excreted (N balance technique) or the change in the total nitrogen in the body.

Biological value

This is the percentage of the *absorbed* nitrogen that is retained in the body (as distinct from the dietary nitrogen). Hence BV is NPU divided by digestibility. Many undamaged protein foods are 90–95% digested, in which case there is little numerical difference between NPU and BV, but this may not be so after heat treatment.

Note that biological value is a specific term although it is sometimes incorrectly used as a synonym for nutritional value.

Protein efficiency ratio – PER

This is the weight gain of the test animals (usually rats) per gram of protein consumed. It has been standardised and is fairly reproducible between laboratories, especially if casein is fed as a standard at the same time and the results corrected for a constant value of 2.5 for casein. The main drawback is that the result is low when less food is eaten if, say, processing or the presence of other substances reduces palatibility, and falsely high if the food is particularly palatable to the animal. Nevertheless it is the most commonly used of the assay methods.

The values range from 4.5 for the highest quality to zero for proteins that cannot support growth when fed as the only source of protein. This does not mean that they have no nutritional value since they can complement other proteins when added to a diet, and PER zero corresponds to NPU 0.4.

Protein efficiency ratio values are not proportional to one another, that is to say PER of 2.0 does not denote a protein twice as useful as one with PER 1.0, whereas a protein with NPU 0.8 has twice as much of the available limiting amino acid as one with NPU 0.4. Thus a fall in PER during processing is indicative of damage but does not reveal much information of the extent of the damage.

Limiting amino acid

The usefulness of a protein for tissue synthesis depends upon its content of that amino acid present in least amount in relation to requirements. This is termed the limiting amino acid. A reduction in nutritional value will only become evident from bioassay if the limiting amino acid is damaged – any damage to an amino acid present in relative surplus will not show up until the damage becomes severe enough to make that amino acid the limiting one.

Lysine is the limiting amino acid in most cereals, and the sulphur amino acids (methionine plus cystine) are limiting in most other foods. Diets as a whole are mostly limited by the S– amino acids.

Complementation

Since the usefulness of a protein depends on that amino acid present in least amount it is possible that two protein sources, each limited by a different amino acid, can have a combined nutritional value superior to either. This is termed complementation.

Detection of nutritional damage

With the highly complex types of reactions that can occur within foods during processing measurement of nutritional change is difficult. Destruction of an amino acid will, of course, be revealed by chemical estimation but we are usually faced with reduced biological availability, which is not revealed chemically.

Estimation of available lysine by fluorodinitrobenzene does not always correlate with biological tests and, for example, can give a high value with raw legumes which have low nutritional value because of the presence of trypsin inhibitors or other toxins.

Even biological tests may not reveal the required information since many of them do not reveal damage to amino acids other than the limiting essential one, and while damage to other amino acids may not be important when the protein is fed alone, it may become so in a mixed diet.

Biological testing with a series of amino acid supplements does provide the required answer but this is an extremely lengthy and expensive procedure. The formation of certain products (indicated by their appearance on a chromatogram of hydrolysed protein) may provide a simpler method of indicating that damage has taken place.

For example, interaction between protein and reducing sugars results in the formation of a lysine-sugar complex which hydrolyses to furosine; alkali damage results in the formation of lysino-alanine, of ornithine from arginine, and of allo-isoleucine.

However, heat damage at near neutral pH results in the formation of internal links between the epsilon-amino groups of lysine and amides which are split during acid hydrolysis of the protein and so leave no trace on the chromatogram. Oxidation leads to the conversion of methionine to the sulphoxide which is destroyed during acid hydrolysis but may be found after alkaline hydrolysis of the protein.

Processing changes

Five types of processing change can be distinguished.

1. The first, which requires only mild heat, is an alteration of the tertiary structure (denaturation) and has no effect on nutritive value. The specific biological properties of the protein molecule, such as enzymic or hormonal activity, are lost. Denaturation is of great importance in food technology since the physical and chemical properties of the proteins are changed. For example, fibrillar proteins can suffer changes in elasticity, flexibility and fibrillar length; globular proteins can suffer changes in solubility, viscosity, osmotic properties, and electrophoretic mobility, among others, that accompany the unfolding of the long chains with the liberation of the reactive groups such as amino, hydroxyl, carboxylic and sulphydryl.

Such changes will alter the properties of the foodstuff, possibly rendering it useless for its normal purpose (for example over-heated wheat gluten has no dough-forming properties) *but have no effect on nutritional value.* After all, boiling an egg or simmering meat will certainly denature the protein, as indeed will the acid of the stomach, but there is no loss of nutritive value.

2. The second type of change is caused by mild heat in the presence of reducing substances and results in a linkage between the end (ε) amino group of lysine with a reducing group, which cannot be hydrolysed by the digestive enzymes. The lysine is still present and is liberated by acid hydrolysis but since it cannot be liberated during digestion it is 'unavailable'. This is the Maillard or non-enzymic browning reaction.

3. More severe heating reduces the availability of other amino acids as well as lysine and can occur in the absence of reducing substances. Cystine is relatively sensitive and can be converted into compounds such as methyl mercaptan, dimethyl sulphide and dimethyl disulphide at temperatures of 115°C. There is usually a fall in digestibility as well.

Reactions can take place within proteins themselves between the free amino groups of lysine and arginine and free acid groups of aspartic and glutamic acids, or with amide groups such as in asparagine and glutamine.

Amino acids can react with sulphur groups, particularly cystine and to a lesser extent methionine, and the imidazole ring of histidine. Phosphodiester links can be formed between two hydroxyamine residues. A lactone ring may be formed between a terminal carboxyl and hydroxyamino acid. Reactions can also take place with fat oxidation products [809].

4. Excessive heat such as applied to the outside of roasted foods leads to

destruction of the amino acids by complete decomposition or by racemisation and the formation of cross-linkages forming polyamino acids [792].
Temperatures of 180-300°C such as are involved in roasting coffee, meat and
fish and in baking of biscuits have these effects. From the nutritional point of
view the D-isomers of the amino acids are not biologically active and they
also have a flavour different from that of the L-isomers. Chemical analysis
reveals destruction of the amino acids.

5. Damage is also caused by alkali treatment and by oxidation. There are
additional factors, possibly but not necessarily, related to nutritive value.
Amino acids are liberated more slowly from damaged proteins – more
nitrogenous compounds are found in the intestine – and this also applies
to raw soybean [818]. This does not necessarily correlate with reduced
digestibility (which would mean reduced nutritive value) but it has been
suggested, without evidence, that the protein might have reduced nutritional value if the amino acids are not all presented simultaneously to the
sites of protein synthesis [810].

The overall biological measurement of net protein utilisation which
includes digestibility would reveal all of these changes – namely, reduced
digestibility, reduced amino acid content or availability and any effect of
slower rates of absorption.

Maillard Reaction

The reaction between lysine and reducing sugars was first observed by
Maillard in 1912 and has been extensively studied (reviewed in detail by
Carpenter and Booth, 1973 [763a]. It is possibly the commonest type of
damage that occurs and even when other amino acids are damaged at the
same time the extent of damage to lysine can be used as an index of the
severity of processing.

The Maillard reaction involves condensation between amino groups of
amino acids in the protein (or in peptide linkage or even free amino acids)
with glycosidic sugars. The first stages of the reaction lead to the formation
of colourless compounds which later complex to form brown pigments,
hence the Maillard reaction is also termed non-enzymic browning. Sulphur
dioxide and other antioxidants can prevent development of the colour but
do not prevent the formation of the colourless amino acid-sugar compounds
and so do not prevent loss of protein quality (Overby et al., 1959). The
kinetics of the browning reaction have been examined by a number of
workers [782, 362, 363], Hodge [795, 899] proposed the reaction scheme
shown in Fig. 4.1.

A variety of groups such as aldehydes, ketones and reducing sugars
combine with amino groups in aldol condensation to form first a Schiff's base

and then an *N*-substituted glycosylamine. These compounds undergo Amadori rearrangement at which stage the compounds formed are still colourless and the reactions are reversible. The third stage is a Strecker degradation with loss of a molecule of carbon dioxide, followed by a condensation of the aldehydes so formed, or condensation with sugar fragments and various dehydration products in the heated food, to form

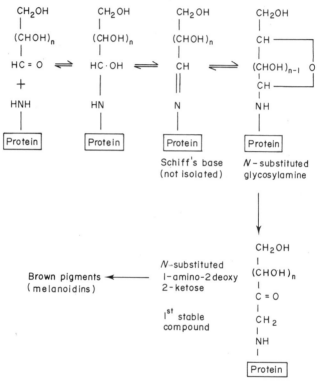

FIG. 4.1. Chemistry of Maillard or browning reaction. (Hodge, 1953 [795]; Finot, 1973 [782])

brown pigments. In the intermediary reactions reductones are formed which interfere with the indophenol method of estimating ascorbic acid.

The first relatively stable compound formed in the Maillard reaction appears to be a 1-deoxy-2-ketose (lysine-fructose) which is not hydrolysed by the digestive enzymes so the lysine is biologically unavailable. Acid hydrolysis liberates half the lysine, forming 20% furosine ((ε-*N*-(2-furoyl-methyl)-L-lysine) and 10% pyridosine (ε-(1,4-dihydro-3-hydroxy-4-oxo-6-methyl-1-pyridyl-L-norleucine) (Fig. 4.2).

On a chromatograph column furosine appears after arginine, and pyridosine before lysine among the basic amino acids.

So the appearance of furosine indicates that part of the lysine has become unavailable. The lysine peak will be partly due to available lysine in the protein and partly due to lysine liberated from lysine-fructose complex.

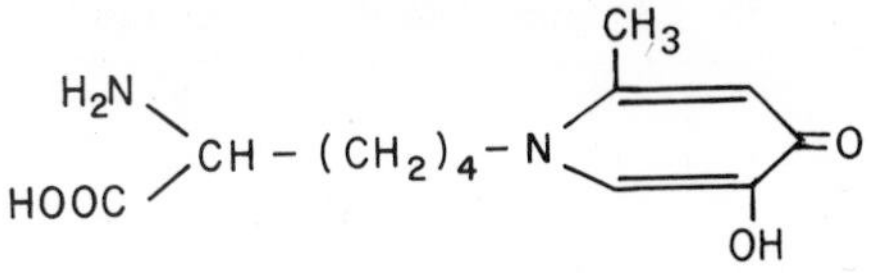

Pyridosine

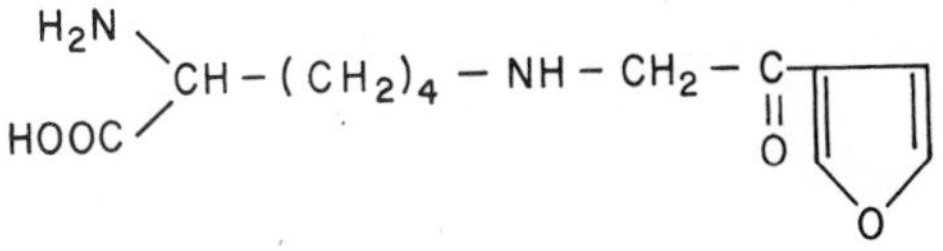

Furosine

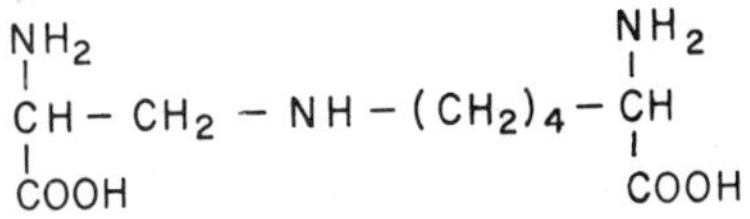

Lysinoalanine

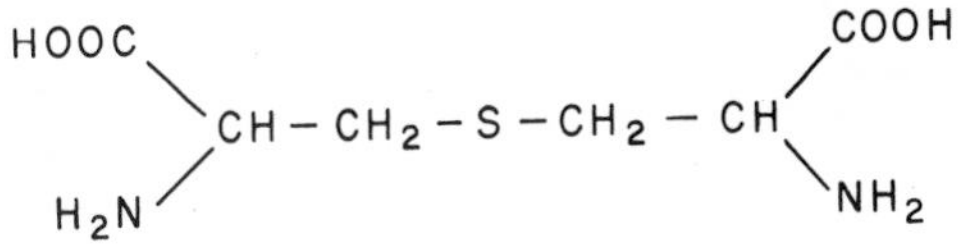

Lanthionine

FIG. 4.2.

Biological assay would be called for [783, 785, 809]. A classical example of the effect of processing was provided by Block *et al.* (1946) [757a]. A cake mix of flour, egg, yeast and lactalbumin had PER 3.5; when baked for 15-20 min at 200°C the value fell to 2.4. Toasting at 130°C for 40-60 min to produce a rusk further reduced PER to 0.8. Damage was solely to lysine since the addition of this amino acid to the toasted product restored the PER to the original value. Similar effects have been shown with a large number of cereal products.

Pronczak *et al.* (1973) [819] compared the laboratory model of casein and glucose heated at 121°C with a product made from wheat flour, sugar, eggs and fat (crisp cake) baked at 180°C for 13 min:

| | | Casein/glucose heated | | | Cake mixture | |
	0	15 min	45 min	135 min	Initial	baked 13 min
NPU	71	67	65	60	74	54
digestibility		95	92	92	87	85
α-amino N in urine	3.4	8.2	9.6	14.6	0	2.0

The authors showed that Maillard compounds were absorbed from the digestive tract and excreted in the urine; digestibility was not affected.

The extent of the Maillard reaction is dependent on a number of factors, as discussed below.

Sulphur amino acids

After lysine, cystine appears to be the next most reactive of the amino acids. Beuk *et al.* (1948) [6, 7] recovered all the amino acids from severely roasted pork except cystine. Bjarnason and Carpenter (1970) [757] heated proteins to 115°C for 27 h (a long period but not an excessive temperature) and destroyed 50% of the cystine. At 145°C almost all the cystine was destroyed but none of the methionine.

While cystine is the most severely damaged of the amino acids in heated soybeans several others can also be damaged. For example, Evans and Butts (1948, 1949) [779, a, b] heated soya meal for 4 h at 121°C with and without sucrose using enzymic *in vitro* digestibility as an index. Without sucrose, when the reactions took place within the protein itself, 37% of the aspartic acid and 24% of the glutamic acid were rendered unavailable. In the presence of sucrose 86% of the cystine, 41% methionine, 47% histidine and 15% of the phenylaline, threonine and leucine were inactivated.

Heat treatment can convert cysteine into cysteic acid, and methionine into methionine sulphone, neither of which is usable. Methionine can also react with fructose to form 1-deoxy-1-methionine-D-fructose [796].

The availability of the sulphur amino acids can be determined biologically by rat assay or by chemical analysis of enzymically hydrolysed protein. Pieniazek *et al.* (1975) [816, 817] carried out the hydrolysis with pancreatopeptidase, then determined the liberated methionine using sodium nitroprusside, which does not react with oxidised forms of methionine. Liberated cysteine and cystine were estimated colorimetrically with dithiobis nitrobenzoic acid.

They showed that the methionine and cysteine were 100% available in pork, beef and fresh whey. Total methionine and cysteine were not changed by processing but availability was reduced (see Table 4.1). Chemical findings were confirmed biologically.

Pieniazek *et al.* (1975) [816] found that like lysine, available methionine in casein was most severely reduced by heating in the presence of both moisture and glucose. Heating dry casein (0.4% moisture) at 90°C for 24 h reduced available methionine by 25%; at 8% moisture it was reduced by 32%. In the presence of glucose the figures were 32% and 55% respectively.

TABLE 4.1. Available sulphur amino acids in fresh and processed food determined after enzymic hydrolysis (Pieniazek *et al.*, 1975 [817])

	Methionine (%)	Cysteine (%)
Fresh milk	100	100
sweetened condensed	85	70
spray dried	100	90*
roller dried	80	90*
Fresh whey	100	100
spray dried	100	100
roller dried	85	100
Fresh mackerel	100	100
steamed	100	100
sterilised at 115°C	100	35
sterilised at 126°C	80	25

* 10% fall in *total* cysteine.

Available cysteine was not affected by moisture, the same losses being found in the dry and the moist casein, namely 60% loss in the absence of glucose and 100% in its presence. Total methionine and cysteine were also reduced but to a smaller extent.

These authors concluded that the fall in the nutritive value of oxidised casein was due not only to oxidation of methionine and cysteine but to the formation within the polypeptide chains of bonds resistant to enzymic hydrolysis. They showed that the formation of cysteic acid in the polypeptide inhibited enzymic release of other adjacent amino acids.

Oxidation

Oxidising agents are used in food processing to a limited extent for a variety of purposes. For example, hydrogen peroxide may be used to sterilise milk, and has been suggested for treatment of yeast and skim milk and to decolourise fish protein concentrate; benzoyl peroxide is used to bleach and improve flour.

At elevated temperatures oxidising agents and also lipid peroxides can react with amino acid residues of proteins and reduce their availability. Methionine is mainly affected forming the sulphoxide which can partially replace methionine in the free state or when peptide bound [767], and the sulphone, which is not usable [776].

Oxidation can result in total destruction of tryptophan and partial destruction of tyrosine. Probably of greater importance is the resistance to enzymic hydrolysis after oxidation. After oxidation with performic acid casein appears to be incompletely hydrolysed *in vivo* judging from animal assay, and enzymic estimation shows reduced availability of proline, glycine, valine, leucine, histidine and arginine [816].

Milk treated with 0.018 M hydrogen peroxide and then hydrolysed with pronase yielded 39% of the total methionine compared with 56% from the untreated food. Half the methionine was oxidised to sulphoxide; other amino acids were not affected [767].

Nitrogen trichloride (agene) once used as a flour improver led to the formation of methionine sulphoximine which caused running fits in dogs.

Hydroperoxides formed from unsaturated fats break down to acids, alcohols and ketones which react with various groupings in proteins [831, 399]. In model systems in which peroxidising methyl linoleate reacted with lysozyme, histamine (from histidine), methionine sulphoxide and various lysine products were formed [799].

Such losses can occur during storage of fatty foods. Carpenter *et al.* (1962) found a decrease of 90% of available lysine in herring meal when stored in air (at 25°C for 12 months) but no change when stored under nitrogen, or when the meal had been defatted [114, 121, 763].

The free radicals produced during lipid oxidation also react with proteins and this effect is reduced by increasing the water content since this quenches the radicals [827].

Since oxidising fats can react with proteins, conversely proteins can function as antioxidants – Labuza *et al.* (1964) found the rate of fat oxidation reduced to one-tenth in the presence of proteins.

Alkali treatment

Protein foods are treated with alkali for a variety of purposes such as destruction of toxins, improvement of functional properties and, in particular, solubilisation in the preparation of protein isolates.

Even mild alkali treatment can reduce nutritional value [112]. At pH above 8 in boiling water or above pH 10 at 25°C cross-linkages can be formed which liberate lysinoalanine on hydrolysis [760]. Apart from nutritional changes this, as discussed below, may be toxic. Among the other changes caused by more severe treatment are the formation of ornithinoalanine by boiling with carbonate, the formation of β-amino alanine by treatment with dilute ammonia or sodium hydroxide, and the loss of or reduced availability of cystine, arginine, threonine, serine, isoleucine and lysine [820]. Lysine, methionine and isoleucine can be racemised and their D-isomers have no nutritional value.

The main compounds formed are lysinoalanaine and lanthionine (Fig. 4.2) (a compound formed from cystine and dehydroalanine [766, 769, 820, 840]).

Damage increases with the severity of treatment. De Groot and Slump (1969) [769] treated soybean protein with alkali at pH 12 for 8 h at 60°C while Woodward and Short (1973) [840] held the temperature at 40°C for 4 h at the same pH. Cystine was generally the most sensitive amino acid. The Net protein utilisation of soya fell from 63 to 41 while that of the isolate (which had been solubilised and precipitated) was as low as 24. The Net protein utilisation of casein was reduced from 63 to 53 and digestibility from 100% to 90%. Treatment of sunflower seed protein with 0.2 N alkali damaged, in order of loss, arginine, threonine, serine, lysine and cystine, with the production of lysinoalanine, alloisoleucine and ornithine and the racemisation of lysine.

Provansal et al. (1975) [766, 820] solubilised proteins in 0.5M NaOH at 55°C for 30 min followed by precipitation with M HCl at pH 4.8 and 4°C; they showed loss of arginine, leucine, cystine, threonine, serine, lysine and isoleucine but no damage to aspartic and glutamic acids, methionine, phenylalanine, proline or tyrosine.

Different proteins respond differently to alkali treatment depending on the number and relative positions of the various reactive groups within the protein. Thus less lysinoalanine was formed in rapeseed protein than in sunflower protein.

The various compounds left after acid hydrolysis of the alkali-damaged protein serve as an index of damage unlike the internal peptide links formed by heating near neutral pH, since these are completely hydrolysed by acid [756].

Apart from loss of nutritional value there is a problem of the possible toxicity of lysinoalanine. The substance itself has been shown to damage the kidneys of the rat (cytomegalia of the straight portion of the proximal tubules) [840] but it does not appear to be harmful when part of the protein complex. Van Beek et al. (1974) [835] did not find any kidney damage after feeding rats with spun soya isolate that had been alkali treated. Moreover, lysinoalanine has been found to be widely distributed in a variety of cooked foods. Sternberg et al. (1975) [829] found amounts ranging from 50 μg/g in some foods to as much as 50 mg/g in a commercial whipping agent. When egg white was fried for 10 min 350 μg lysinoalanine was produced per g egg white and a commercially dried sample contained 1.8 mg/g. Evaporated milks used in infant formulae contained 150 to 860 μg/g and soya isolate contained 0–370 μg/g. Hence lysinoalanine appears to be formed even by heat alone.

Other factors

A number of carbonyl compounds used in processing react with fish protein (used for animal feed) in the dry form by reducing the amount of available lysine, and in aqueous solution by promoting cross-linkages within the protein; e.g. formaldehyde, acetal, and propional [122].

Formaldehyde reacts with proteins and protects them from hydrolysis and degradation by bacteria in the rumen of cattle and this treatment actually improves their nutritional value for ruminants.

Cottonseed contains a pigment gossypol and during processing of the seed to obtain the oil part of this combines with the free amino groups of lysine reducing its availability [765].

Solvents used in fat extraction can damage the protein. Fish meals processed for human consumption (fish flours and fish protein concentrates) are often extracted with solvent. Ethanol [130] and isopropanol do not damage the protein unless temperatures of 100–120°C are used over a period of several hours [119]. A grade of high aldehyde content did result in reduction of available lysine.

However, the solvent 1,2-dichlorethane reacts with cysteine and methionine to form toxic compounds [131, 132]. McKinney et al. (1957) [806] showed that cysteine was converted into S-(dichlorovinyl)-L-cysteine which was toxic to calves.

Factors controlling processing damage

The principal factors affecting the protein-sugar reactions were established by the classic study of Lea and Hannan (1949) [801]. They mixed sodium caseinate in water with 11% glucose and freeze-dried the mixture so that there was intimate contact between the protein and the sugar. Storage at 37°C resulted in maximum loss of reactive amino groups when the moisture content was between 15 and 18% i.e. 70% relative humidity. The reaction was retarded at low pH – the rate at pH 3 was one-tenth of that at pH 7 – but only slightly accelerated at alkaline pH.

The loss of reactive amino groups was confirmed biologically by Henry and Kon (1950) on the same material [793]; after 30 days the loss of 90% of the reactive amino groups was accompanied by a fall in BV from 0.78 to 0.39 (this final value approximates to the values found with mixtures of amino acids completely lacking lysine) the digestibility of the mixture was still 91% of the initial value.

The amino acid mostly, affected varies with the food and the conditions. Casein-glucose mixtures and cereal products suffer damage to lysine alone with relatively mild heat. More severe heat begins to damage sulphur amino acids and to a lesser extent others. Materials such as meat meals and fish meals that have been heated severely suffer damage mainly to S-amino acids.

Moisture

Lea and Hannan (1949) [801] established that damage is most severe at 10% and 14% moisture (70% relative humidity). Carpenter *et al.* (1962) [114] found that the loss of available lysine was greatest at 4 to 14% moisture. Dry materials are relatively resistant to heat [127] and boiling in excess water has no effect.

Skimmed milk powder was stored at 4.7% moisture for 182 days and suffered no change in BV or digestibility. At 7.3% moisture there was a fall from BV 0.84 to 0.69 after only 60 days (183 184). Milk powder is always stored below 5% moisture to avoid deterioration of qualities such as flavour and solubility and this would appear to be the limit for protein damage also.

Kramer (1974) [902] reported that to keep losses below 10% PER for 6 months requires a temperature of $-1°C$ at RH 60%, but at RH 40% the temperature can be $10°C$. Longer periods of storage require lower temperatures but, contrary to the findings reported above, he stated that there is no significant loss of protein quality after 2 years storage if the temperature is maintained at $-15°C$.

Reducing substances

One of the major factors involved in loss of nutritive value, especially with mild heating, is the presence of reducing sugars. Casein heated alone is stable up to $120°C$ [789] while the casein-glucose mixture of Lea and Hannan was unstable even at $10°C$. Similarly a sample of wheat gluten was stable when heated alone but when glucose was added the BV fell from 0.55 to 0.18 [791]. Baking a biscuit supplemented with casein did not result in any loss of available lysine but when skim milk powder was used instead, the lactose caused a 50% loss of available lysine [237].

Apparent discrepancies in experimental findings may be due to the relative purity of materials used. For example, Mader *et al.* (1949) [805] found that commercial lactalbumin contained 5% reducing sugar and that when this was washed out the protein was less susceptible to heat damage. Similarly washed casein is more stable than a sample contaminated with lactose.

Very small quantities of reducing substances are capable of causing damage, as evidenced by the deterioration of dried egg during storage. There is only 1.2% glucose present, but when this is removed the egg becomes stable [509]. Tarr (1954) [832] showed that the small amount of ribose present in certain species of fish (0.4% of the dry weight) was sufficient to cause protein damage. Carpenter *et al.* (1962) showed that while plasma albumin was unaffected by heating to 85°C for 27 h, the addition of small amounts of ribose caused damage in 1 h at the same temperature. These authors calculated that 0.8 moles of lysine combined with 1 mole ribose (0.3% ribose reacted with 2% lysine) [763b].

Different reducing sugars react at different rates, the fastest being xylose followed in order by arabinose, glucose and galacturonic acid, lactose, maltose and fructose. Fructose was about one-tenth as reactive as glucose [871].

The damaging effect of sucrose and other non-reducing sugars has been explained by suggesting that they are first split to reducing sugars during processing [763b]. For example sucrose does not react with casein but markedly increases the loss of available lysine from heated soya bean isolate [779a] and groundnut isolate [398]. Sucrose caused a loss of lysine in baked biscuits when its concentration was 29% but not at 14.5% [236].

Amino acids can react with reducing substances formed by oxidation of fats in the food. Tappel (1955) [831] used model systems of linoleic acid or cod liver oil emulsified with protein and oxidative catalyst. After 48 h at 37°C there was extensive interaction between protein and oxidising fat with the formation of insoluble dark brown compounds and destruction of amino acids.

Lea *et al.* (1958) [121] found a smaller effect in herring meal. This absorbed oxygen within a few weeks at 37°C, more slowly at 25°C. Available lysine fell only from 7.2 g/16 g N to 6.6 in 12 months storage at 25°C (6 or 11% moisture in the meal). There was no loss of available lysine when the meal was either stored in nitrogen or defatted before storing in air. Thus the loss of lysine was associated, as found by Tappel [831], with oxidation of the oil. Although methionine can be oxidised, feeding trials by these same authors showed that the only damage was to the lysine.

Time/temperature

Reduction of protein quality can take place at room temperature i.e. it can occur during storage. The severe loss of quality in the casein-glucose mixture described above took place at 37°C. Ben-Gera and Zimmerman (1972) [755] stored various materials at temperatures up to 40°C and 60% RH in closed bags in partial vacuum and found the following maximum losses of available lysine: skim milk powder 88%, cottonseed meal 36%, groundnut meal 33%, chickpeas 30%, wheat 43%, rice 19%, sorghum 40% and soybean meal 8%.

The acceleration of damage by heat can be most marked. Lea and Hannan (1949) [801] found that the reaction of their model system proceeded at a measurable rate at 10°C, was 100 times faster at 37°C and 9000 times faster at 70°C. When proteins are heated alone they are generally stable up to a critical temperature beyond which damage is proportional to temperature and time. Casein, for example, was not damaged until the temperature reached 120°C, above that the damage was proportional to the time of heating [789]. Even in the presence of reducing sugars, short mild heat treatment sometimes has little effect – casein autoclaved with glucose (ratio 50 : 1) at 121°C showed a small fall in digestibility from 95% to 92% after 135 min; NPU fell to 95% of the original value after 15 min, 92% after 45 min and 85% after 135 min [819]. These losses are in marked contrast to those shown by Lea and Hannan described above.

Mauron *et al.* (1960) [270] found that the losses in high-protein biscuits were proportional to time and temperature as were the model systems. Pronczuk *et al.* (1973) [819] examined biscuits subjected to 180°C for 13 min, when NPU fell to 72% of the original value.

Carpenter and Booth (1973) have produced an Arrhenius plot showing rate of loss of reactive amino groups at different temperatures [763a].

Other factors

Many of the investigations of protein stability have been carried out on model systems but foodstuffs are much more complicated than casein-glucose models, and there appear to be additional factors that can affect protein quality.

Dummer (1971) [773] found that a heated casein-glucose mixture lost arginine, threonine, methionine, histidine and isoleucine in that order, as well as lysine but when milk was heated under the same conditions only lysine was lost.

Physical factors are likely to be involved. For example Bender (unpublished) found that diets for experimental animals composed largely of glucose and casein were quite stable in open containers at room temperature even after a year, in marked contrast to the rapid loss of quality at room temperature reported by Lea and Hannan.

A factor that will be obvious to every process engineer is that the temperature of importance is that reached by the food not the heating medium. For example there are many reports of little or no damage to fish meal in flame dryers where the inlet temperature was 1100°C. There were charred residues on the hot ducts but the quality of the meal was relatively good. This is simply due to the fact that the temperature of the food cannot rise above 100°C until all the water has been removed so that it is possible that the fish meal itself never reached a high temperature. Conversely, there have been many failed attempts to produce undamaged materials despite carefully controlled processing conditions.

The anomalies can be illustrated by the relative instability of a sample of dried milk (only one sample was examined) stored under apparently perfect conditions – under nitrogen and in deep freeze [751]. After 3 years the NPU had fallen from 0.74 to 0.53. What is even more inexplicable is that another sample, after being assayed, had been left open in the store cupboard for the same length of time exposed to atmospheric temperatures and humidity and had set to a solid mass. This unprotected material had the same NPU as the sample carefully stored. In both samples the damage was incurred by the sulphur amino acids since the addition of methionine restored the NPUs to 0.73.

Physiological effects of Maillard compounds

Nutritionally, protein quality is reduced when some portion of an essential amino acid is rendered unavailable but there may be other effects [747b].

1. Failure to hydrolyse amino acid linkages reduces digestibility and leads to the excretion of peptide fragments in the faeces.

2. Alternatively, some unhydrolysed peptides are absorbed from the intestine (i.e. they are 'digested') but they are excreted in the urine. This explains why some workers have observed a greater fall in nutritive value than could be accounted for by reduced digestibility of the protein [788, 819].

3. The rate of release of amino acids from heated proteins may be delayed so altering their usefulness for protein synthesis.

4. Undigested peptides in the intestine interfere with absorption of amino acids by partial inhibition of the digestive enzymes [803] and also inhibition of the amino acid transport system from the digestive tract. Adami and Hewitt (1975) [395] found this effect with isolated intestinal cells. Lee *et al.* (1976) [803] showed that heating tryptophan with glucose gave rise to fructose-L-tryptophan which competitively inhibited the absorption of tryptophan (as shown by the everted sac technique). To consider a more practical product, severely browned apricot caused diarrhoea (to which

animals adapted), and reduced growth rate on constant food intake. There was also evidence of liver damage, deduced from changes in the levels of various enzymes.

Tanaka *et al.* (1976) [829a] showed that damaged protein depressed the activities of disaccharidases, alkaline phosphatase and some dipeptidases in the intestinal mucosa, increased the lipid content of the liver, and enhanced the activity of hepatic transaminase. This damaged protein was not the result of severe overheating but simply produced by storing egg albumin with glucose at 37°C and 68% RH. After 10 days there was a fall in BV without the appearance of a brown colour (which appeared later). Lysine and arginine were the amino acids affected.

5. It has been stated that that the products of the Maillard reaction are toxic [747b, 748] but the situation is not clear. It has been pointed out that soluble material extracted from Maillard-reacted foods behaves differently from the material in protein complex [759, 782]. The soluble complex of fructose-lysine is absorbed from the intestine and excreted in the urine but it is not absorbed from protein foods.

However, Ford and Shorrock (1971) [788] and Pronczuk *et al.* (1973) [819] found compounds of large molecular weight in the urine of animals fed heated casein-glucose mixtures. Direct feeding trials with heated cod-glucose and egg white-glucose did not depress rat growth nor did severely overheated milk preparations fed to infants.

Desirable browning

The Maillard reaction can make a positive contribution to food technology by producing desirable colours, flavours and aromas. E.g. in baking, roasting, frying and toasting, such as in biscuits, breakfast cereals, roasted peanuts, cocoa, meat extract, and malt extract [267, 747a]. Although there is some loss of amino acids when these flavours are produced this is usually small and is accepted as a price worth paying. The Maillard reaction can be exploited for particular purposes by the addition of reducing agents to the food. For example, the inclusion of milk powder in bread permits more even toasting at a lower temperature because of the presence of lactose.

Another example is the production of chicken and meat-like flavours by heating amino acids with pentose sugars and aldehydes. Cysteine and ribose produce a pork-like flavour, ribose with a mixture of amino acids produces a beef-like flavour, lysine or cystine with furan produces meat-flavour. The specific flavours of breakfast cereals, baked bread, roasted coffee and soya flour are said to be due to the reaction of particular amino acids. Glucose heated with glycine gives the flavour of freshly baked bread, with amino butyric acid it gives a maple syrup flavour, methionine breakdown products have the flavour of potato [794, 838]. Adrian (1973) gives a table of flavours produced by different amino acids and sugars [747a].

The volatile products from cooked vegetables are aldehydes derived from amino acids such as alanine, valine, leucine, etc. The less pleasant flavours are associated with Strecker degradation products of sulphur-containing amino acids (methyl mercaptan, dimethylsulphide, methylsulphide, etc.).

Rao (1974) [458] examined groundnut meal and Bengal gram (Indian multipurpose food) that had been heated to improve the flavour. It was necessary to heat to at least 120°C to produce an attractive flavour but the sucrose present in the groundnut resulted in considerable damage:

Heating (min)	Loss of thiamin	Riboflavin	Change in PER
10	50%	10%	fall from 1.75 to 1.55
20	60%	30%	fall from 1.75 to 1.55
30	70%	40%	fall from 1.75 to 1.42

The fall in PER was due to reduced available lysine, the values being, respectively 3.0, 2.5 and 1.7% of protein at the three time periods.

Bengal gram lost 85% of the riboflavin and all of the thiamin after 10 min heating; PER fell from 1.7 to 1.5 due to a reduction in available lysine from 6.1 to 3.5%.

Relevance to practical diets

Nearly all the investigations discussed in this chapter were carried out on rats and the results extrapolated to human beings. This appears to be quite illogical since it is known that there are considerable differences between the two in relative rates of growth and maintenance and therefore in the ratios of the amino acids required. However, in practice the lysine requirements of the baby approximate to those of the growing rat and the few proteins that have been examined on both species have given similar results [754].

It is not at all clear how far rat assays can be applied to adult human beings. Cereals for example, according to the limited amount of information available from human experiments, appear to differ for the two species. The BV of whole wheat measured on the rat has been variously reported as 0.64, 0.67, 0.68 and 0.76; while one laboratory reported values for man of 0.90 for shredded whole wheat and toasted whole wheat, and 0.80 for puffed and flaked wheat. The results at least confirm that there is damage to the wheat protein on processing.

Oats have NPU 0.66 for rat and 0.89 for man, wheat germ 0.75 for rat and 0.89 for man; on the other hand wheat gluten appears to be 0.40 for both species [754].

It is not known whether these discrepancies are real differences between the two species, or due to the errors inherent in the small number of difficult determinations that have been carried out in man compared with the many replications of rat assays. Certainly Calloway and Margen (1971) found that the BV of egg protein measured in human subjects varied between 0.46 and 0.81, so there may well be considerable individual variation or variation in the same individual from time to time.

However, while it is not clear whether nutritional values as determined on experimental animals are applicable to man, laboratory experimentation does demonstrate whether and where there has been processing damage. Moreover, if absolute results are not required (and from what has been said above they may not be applicable to man) and quality control is the issue, then almost any of the tests discussed will be adequate.

Chapter 5

CARBOHYDRATES

Compared with labile nutrients such as vitamins, carbohydrates are generally regarded as being completely stable to processing. However there is some loss both by leaching into processing water and by breakdown but since this is 'merely' a loss of energy as distinct from nutrients it is usually disregarded.

Losses by leaching will be governed by the same factors that affect other water-soluble materials as discussed elsewhere – particle size, time, volume of water, etc.

Losses by breakdown are exemplified by the cooking of broad beans [465]. during preliminary soaking there was a decrease in starch and an increase in sugars. During baking (120°C for 150 min) there was a decrease in total carbohydrates and in protein and amino acids through combination to form brown pigments. Sugar content fell from 10.8% to 9.3%; starch content fell from 34% to 31%, being converted first into dextrins then into reducing sugars. Such a change from one carbohydrate to another involves no loss and can be a gain if digestibility of the carbohydrate is increased by the treatment.

Overheating can lead to the formation of unpalatable products; for example at sterilising temperatures substances such as laevulinic acid, reductones and 5-hydroxymethylfurfural can be formed, leading to coloured products. This would not involve any significant loss of nutritional value.

MINERAL SALTS

Inorganic salts are completely stable but can be leached out into water. Although such losses are usually disregarded they can be considerable. For example McCance *et al.* (1936) [360] and Krehl and Winters (1950) [354] showed losses of 12–40% of the calcium of carrots, beans, cabbage and other vegetables, together with 60% of the potassium chloride.

Methods of cooking, volume of water, surface-to-volume ratio and the various factors discussed under Blanching control the amounts lost. Saito (1069) [845] found a loss of 32% of the iron and 9% of the calcium from a variety of foods when cooked by Japanese methods but these losses were only 17 and 5% respectively when 'European methods' were used. Kizlaitis *et al.* (1964) showed small losses of iron among other minerals from cooked meats [47].

It is the gain in minerals from processing and cooking water that may be of greater importance in certain instances. For example, low-sodium foods are required in a variety of disorders and care has to be taken to avoid the pick-up of sodium from the water [847]. Drinking water may contain up to 10 mg sodium per 100 cm^3 which can be increased to 50 mg by softening. In canned foods sodium, and other solutes, tends to distribute itself uniformly between the food and the liquid. In one series of observations the sodium content of garden peas increased from 1.7 to 12 mg per 100 g on canning. Brining used to prevent discolouration of vegetables or for quality grading leaves sodium on the product even after rinsing. In one report an initial level in garden peas of 1.2 mg per 100 g increased to 8–18 mg after 'light brining' and rinsing, and to 36 mg after 'heavy brining'.

Lye peeling and the use of sodium salts as processing aids and additives may increase the mineral content of the food. Iron can be picked up from plant machinery and, in fact, accounts for the greater part of the iron content of curry spices.

Gurevič (1966) [118] reported a considerable loss of iodide from herring. This amounted to 50–100% on freezing and almost all was lost when samples of dog salmon, smelt, herring, plaice, cod and rudd were defrosted and refrozen. heavy salting caused 30–40% loss and hot smoking 30%; light salting and cold smoking caused smaller losses.

LIPIDS

Lipids undergo a number of degradative changes which have a much greater effect on palatability than upon their nutritional value. The nutritional value of fats is limited to the energy content of the triglycerides and to their content of essential fatty acids. Some fats contain vitamins in solution and it is damage to them and to the essential fatty acids that constitute any problems relating to loss of nutritional value.

An additional factor is the fall in protein quality following reaction between breakdown products of the fats and amino acids, as discussed under Proteins, p. 70.

Changes in the fat content of the food itself must be included under nutritional changes – some foods may gain fat and so increase their energy content, and possibly their EFA and vitamin content, others may lose fat in the process.

A problem with calculations of nutrient changes arises from loss of fats as it does with loss of water in processing. For example, there is a considerable loss of fat when bacon is cooked, leading to an increase in nutrients calculated per 100 g dry weight, which may show as a loss if calculated per 100 g protein.

Chemical changes

Fats can readily undergo peroxidation by autoxidation, by chemical catalysis and by enzymic catalysis with lipoxidase (lipoxygenase) naturally present or from microbial contamination. These changes take place relatively slowly so that quality deteriorates during prolonged storage rather than suffering any sudden loss during processing. An exception to this generalisation is the damage during frying if the temperature is allowed to rise excessively. As described later there is limited damage under controlled frying conditions but this can be cumulative if the same fat is used repeatedly.

Oxidative and hydrolytic breakdown can spoil the flavour of a food even when the fats are present in very small amounts, e.g. vegetables such as potatoes, spinach and beans contain as little as 0.1 to 0.6% fat but this is sufficient to cause deterioration of flavour during storage. Unsaturated fats are more liable to oxidation.

Autoxidation starts with the formation of hydroperoxides catalysed by traces of metals, particularly copper, and by haematin compounds, and is accelerated by light, heat and radiation of various types. The reaction propagates a chain reaction leading to the formation of alkyl hydroperoxides which break down to short chain aldehydes, ketones and acids and form polymers with unpleasant rancid flavours.

During peroxide formation free radicals are produced which react with proteins and vitamins, as well as enzymes and with other lipids. Vitamin A is particularly susceptible to damage by peroxidation. Protection is effected by antioxidants which appear to function by reacting rapidly with free radicals and so preventing further spread of the chain reaction.

Plant materials especially peas, beans, cereal grains and oil seeds contain the enzyme lipoxidase, which gives rise to hydroperoxides. This enzyme is specific for fatty acids with cis-cis methylene interrupted diene structure i.e. the fatty acids such as linoleic acid, and so could lead to nutritional damage. However, the food becomes unpalatable before nutritional changes become significant so the normal practice of ensuring destruction of such enzymes as an essential part of food processing would automatically provide protection of the nutrient in this particular respect.

Moisture can influence oxidative susceptibility in two different directions – it may promote or inhibit. In cereal products low moisture favours rancidity development, but low moisture in dried egg and dried milk (less than 2%) is protective.

Heat treatment obviously destroys the enzyme but autoxidation can continue even in the cold and is the reason for quality deterioration in frozen foods containing fat and for the potential loss of the fat soluble vitamins during cold storage.

At the high temperatures employed in frying breakdown is much more rapid and a range of volatile carbonyls, hydroxyacids, ketoacids, epoxy acids and oxipolymers are formed. Polymerisation can take place in the absence of oxygen to yield cyclic compounds and higher polymers. These latter compounds have been implicated in the toxicity of heated fats [853, 875, 877].

The effects of lipid degradation thus fall under three headings; (1) formation of unpalatable compounds; (2) the possible formation of toxic compounds; (3) reduction of nutritive value. Also, the addition or removal of fat from the food during processing must be taken into account.

Nutritional changes

Two points emerge from this discussion in which lipids differ from other food ingredients – there is little, if any, immediate loss of nutritional value on processing, and deterioration can continue at low temperatures.

Most experimental evidence indicates no significant loss of nutritional value in normal heat processing of fatty foods such as dairy products, and eggs [153, 203] and meat fats cooked either conventionally or by microwave [14, 67]. Baking has little or no effect [99, 278].

Low temperatures usually enable foods to be stored for long periods since the components are stable but fats can still be oxidised at these temperatures. Owen et al. (1975) [73] showed that the rancidity of stored pork was partly due to the oxidation of polyunsaturated fatty acids taking place while frozen. Poultry fat is less saturated than beef or lamb and less stable; its stability can be enhanced by feeding extra tocopherol to the chickens [100, 869].

In particular, as discussed under vitamin E, hydroperoxides which break down at room temperature are stable at low temperatures and react with and destroy more of the tocopherols during frozen storage than at room temperature.

Vitamins – retinol, carotenoids, cholecalciferol and tocopherols – present in fats and oils undergo oxidation while the fat itself is being oxidised. The preferential oxidation of tocopherols confers on them the properties of antioxidants and they are present, and function as such, in many vegetable oils. They are also added to fats and fatty foods for this purpose and, as mentioned elsewhere, can be fed to chickens to serve as antioxidants in the body fat. Their effectiveness as antioxidants is obviously accompanied by their destruction, although of the various tocopherols naturally present in foods those with the highest antioxidant properties have lower relative vitamin potencies.

Ascorbyl palmitate is also added as an antioxidant and acts synergistically with the tocopherols, but the amounts of both these vitamins added are too small to make any significant contribution to nutritional intake.

The losses of vitamins in oxidising fats are discussed under the individual vitamins.

Polyunsaturated fatty acids

Certain types of polyunsaturated fatty acids are dietary essentials since they cannot be synthesised in the body; these are termed the essential fatty acids, EFA, and were at one time called vitamin F. The group comprises linoleic, linolenic and arachidonic acids. The first two are found in vegetable oils and can be converted in the animal body into arachidonic acid so the name EFA applies to them.

It is the *cis-cis* methylene interrupted isomer that appears to be the dietary essential so either oxidation of the double bonds or isomerisation results in a loss of nutritive properties.

In practice a dietary deficiency of EFA never seems to occur, probably because the requirement is so small, about 1 g per day, so processing damage would not appear to be a significant factor in this respect.

However, there appear to be other nutritional properties of polyunsaturated fatty acids – PUFA – (both EFA and others such as $C_{20:5}$ and $C_{22:6}$ found in marine oils). They are implicated in the highly complex problem of diet, blood cholesterol levels and ischaemic heart disease. This is not the place even to outline the facts and theories postulated but there is evidence that a ratio of polyunsaturated fatty acids to saturated of $2:1$ in the diet is effective in lowering plasma cholesterol levels, which may, in turn, reduce the risk factor in heart disease. Hence any loss of PUFA is, in a sense, a reduction in nutritional properties. Moreover, saturated fatty acids such as palmitic and myristic elevate cholesterol levels, while stearic acid and middle chain triglycerides have little effect. Thus processing may affect nutritional value by altering the types and ratios of fatty acids in a food.

The refining of oils has no nutritional effect although it does remove the phytosterols which have been shown to lower blood cholesterol. However, the amounts present in the crude oils are probably too small to have any beneficial effect.

Hydrogenation can both saturate the polyunsaturates and also cause isomerisation with consequent loss of biological activity.

The high temperatures employed in frying would be expected to destroy a large part of such apparently labile compounds as polyunsaturated carbon chains but in practice, the losses are small, probably because of the natural antioxidant content, apart from those added commercially.

Kilgore and Bailey (1970) [866] simulated practical conditions by frying chipped potatoes in various vegetable oils and re-using the same oil for several repeat operations. They use a standardised size of chipped potatoes (0.5×0.25×4.5 inches) fried for 12 min at 185±5°C. Four half pound batches were fried each day, with a 10 min gap between batches and allowing the oils to cool to 9°C overnight. The process was repeated on each of 5 successive days so that finally 10 lb of potato chips had been fried in the same batch of oil – total heating time 7.5 h. The results are shown in Table 5.].

TABLE 5.1. Linoleic acid in oils after frying (as % of total fatty acids) (Kilgore and Bailey, 1970 [866])

		Safflower oil[1]	Corn[2]	Cottonseed[3]	Vegetable shortening[4]
Initial		72	57	56	30
After frying	2 lb	71	56	54	29
	4 lb	72	56	51	29
	6 lb	70	54	52	28
	8 lb	70	53	50	27
	10 lb	70	51	49	27

[1] With added antioxidants BHA, BHT, propyl gallate, citric acid and propylene glycol. [2] With isopropyl citrate and methyl silicone. [3] No additive. [4] Methyl silicone only.

Not until 6 lb of potatoes had been fried did the reduction in linoleic acid content become significant, but even these changes were small; safflower oil was unchanged even after frying 10 lb of potatoes but this had a battery of antioxidants added. Cottonseed oil with no added antioxidants lost only 10% of its initial linoleic acid content.

The fat extracted from the fried potato chips showed slightly greater falls in linoleic acid content (Table 5.2) for cottonseed and safflower oils but not the other two.

The authors themselves regard these small differences between the oil and the food as being significant and suggest that branched chain compounds and unstable peroxide-linked polymers may have been formed but not absorbed by the potatoes, or that oxidation may have occurred in the food on the surface after processing before analysis.

While it might be expected that the more highly unsaturated safflower oil would show greater instability this was apparently overcome by the added antioxidants.

At higher temperatures there is, as would be expected, greater destruction of linoleic acid but it is still not very marked. The results of Fleischman *et al.* (1963) [859] can be used for purposes of comparison with those of Kilgore and Bailey. They fried chipped potatoes both at 190°C, when their results agreed well with those described above, and also at 257°C.

At the lower temperature there was only a small fall in the polyenoic acid content of corn oil in three successive batches, namely from 67% of the total fatty acids to 63%, 61% and 62%.

In the experiment at the higher temperature it took 30 min to reach 257°C then 50 min to cool to 66°C, with the following results:

(*a*) safflower oil: polyenoic acids fell from 91% to 78% of the total fatty acids, (*b*) corn oil: from 67% to 42%, (*c*) peanut oil: from 41% to 36%, and

TABLE 5.2. Linoleic acid extracted from fried potatoes (as % of total fatty acid) (Kilgore and Bailey, 1970 [866])

	Safflower oil	Corn	Cottonseed	Shortening
1st lb fried	71	57	54	29
2nd	73	57	54	30
3rd	71	56	53	29
4th	71	56	52	29
5th	70	54	51	29
6th	70	55	52	28
7th	65	56	52	28
8th	66	55	52	27
9th	67	51	48	27
10th	65	50	43	27

(*d*) soybean oil: from 62% to 50%. Similar measurements of changes in EFA content of the food and the frying oil are discussed under Poultry; [871].

Under controlled factory conditions processing temperatures can be kept at the minimum required, but under uncontrolled domestic conditions much higher temperatures may be reached. Fleischman *et al.* (1963) [859] also examined oils used only once under the following conditions and reported much greater losses than in the chipped potatoes.

1. *Domestic*: frying 3 large potatoes in corn oil 15 min at 205°C – fall of polyenoic acid from 67% to 54%.
2. *Hospital*: frying chicken for $2\frac{1}{2}$ h at 191°C in cottonseed oil – fall from 66% to 35%.
3. *Hospital*: frying chicken for 1 h and then potatoes for $\frac{1}{2}$ h at 191°C – fall from 66% to 58%.
4. Corn fritters heated 3 h at 191°C – fall from 66% to 55%.

Clearly surface area, time, temperature and food lipids and other constituents will affect the loss of polyunsaturated fatty acids.

Alteration of fatty acid composition

While not strictly within the concept of changes wrought by a manufacturing process the feeding of polyunsaturates to animals with the intention of altering the composition of their body fat might be worthy of inclusion.

It is obviously possible to manufacture foods rich in polyunsaturated fats simply by replacing the normal fats with the desired type. Red meats and dairy produce, however, often provide half the fat intake in the western world and nearly three quarters of the saturated fats. Feeding polyunsaturated fats to cattle is not effective in altering their body fat since they are hydrogenated in the rumen, and they must reach the abomasum unchanged. A method of overcoming the problem was introduced by Cook *et al.* [856, 857, 879] by spray-drying a mixture of the vegetable oil (safflower in this instance) with casein and coating the product with formaldehyde. This complex is not digested by the bacteria of the rumen and reaches the abomasum. When fed to lambs at 20% of the dietary intake there was an increase in the linoleic acid content of the carcass – in mesenteric fat the level increased from 1.9% of the total fat to 11% after 3 weeks and 16% after 6 weeks feeding. Milk fat can also be altered similarly.

Margarines

One of the commonest and richest sources of polyunsaturated fatty acids in the diet is margarine made from the appropriate fats. During the hydrogenation of the oils isomerisation can occur with loss of biological activity, e.g. from the *cis-cis* isomer to *cis-trans, trans-cis* or *trans-trans*. However, there are methods of hydrogenation which avoid this and margarines are manufactured which are both rich in the active polyunsaturates and free from *trans* isomers.

Chapter 6

STABILITY OF ADDED NUTRIENTS

Many processed foods are enriched by a variety of nutrients – vitamins, amino acids, mineral salts and proteins, see chapter 9.

The stability of added nutrients may differ from those naturally present, partly because of possible differences in their chemical form but perhaps largely because of the physical protection afforded to the natural nutrients by the other food ingredients. At the same time stabilised forms of vitamins are used which may be more stable than those naturally present.

Consequently added nutrients can be more stable or less stable than the natural ones. Shemer and Perkins (1975) [467] showed that added methionine was more sensitive than the methionine present in protein combination in enriched soya, as did Carnovale *et al.* (1969) [230] who compared the stability of amino acids added to soya flour and subjected to extrusion cooking. In a semolina pasta 7% of the total lysine and 7% of the threonine of the protein were destroyed compared with 25% of the added lysine, 14% of the added threonine and 18% of the added methionine. These values were determined chemically so any reduction in availability is not known.

One of the methods of enriching whole grain cereal with amino acids is to soak the scarified grain in the nutrient solution. This was done by Tara and Bains (1971) [297] who cooked rice in a solution of lysine and threonine so that the entire solution was absorbed into the grains. After this treatment milled rice needed boiling for 14 min to become edible and there was no loss of amino acids; parboiled rice required 28 min cooking and the loss was 5% of the amino acids, probably within the limits of accuracy of estimation.

Treatment more severe than boiling can damage added lysine [222]. Lysine in maize was increased tenfold by soaking in a solution and when the maize was subsequently 'popped' 40% of this was destroyed.

In bread [258] and in biscuits [236] added lysine has the same degree of stability as that naturally present.

Vitamins can be prepared in protected forms coated with gelatin, starch or shellac and vitamins added to cereal grains or flours may be more stable than those naturally present. For example, Cort *et al.* (1976) [240] prepared a premix of vitamin A, thiamin mononitrate, riboflavin, niacin, pyridoxine hydrochloride, folic acid, reduced iron and tocopherol acetate in starch that was stable for 6 months when stored at room temperature in polythene bags. When blended with wheat flour at 9% moisture together with a mineral salt premix, all the vitamins except vitamin A were completely stable for 6 months at room temperature and 12 weeks at 45°C, 15% of the vitamin A was lost after 8 weeks and 25% after 12 weeks storage.

At the higher moisture content of 13.5%, which is more usual, 10% of the vitamin A was lost in 4 weeks at 45°C but pyridoxine, tocopherol and folate were stable. These three vitamins were also completely stable to baking (the other vitamins were not measured).

Similarly all added vitamins except A were stable in yellow corn meal stored 6 months at room temperature. After 12 weeks at 45°C 30% of the vitamin A was lost. This, according to the authors, is equivalent to 2.5 years at room temperature.

Rice was enriched with a complete range of vitamins protected with either zein-stearic acid-shellac or with ethyl cellulose and shellac. After 6 months at room temperature vitamins A and E were stable, and 10% of the folate and B_6 were lost. On cooking there was a loss of less than 10% of the vitamin A and no loss of B_6, folate and E (thiamin was not measured).

Bunting (1965) showed that pyridoxine added to corn meal was stable for 1 year at 38°C and 50% RH and also stable to baking [226].

Cording et al. (1961) [480] examined the stability of natural and added vitamin C in potato flakes, prepared by cooking, mashing, drum drying and flaking. There was 30% loss of both natural and added vitamin C during the process and another 30% loss after 28 weeks storage at 24°C and 5% moisture. This loss took place even when antioxidants were included but not when the product was stored under nitrogen.

Added thiamin was completely destroyed because of the presence of sulphite but added water-dispersible vitamin A, riboflavin and niacin were stable to processing and to storage.

Bender (1958) [313] found the same degree of stability for added vitamin C as for that naturally present in a fruit squash stored for periods up to 2 years.

Keagy et al. (1975) [259] found that folate added as pteroyl glutamic acid to flour was more stable to storage than the naturally occurring vitamin. Flour containing 0.12 μg/g natural folic acid stored at 12.5% moisture lost 15% in 2 months at 29°C and 40% at 49°C. After that it was stable for one year. Folate added at 1 to 5 μg/g flour was stable for 1 year at both 29°C and 38°C. At the higher temperature of 49°C there was a loss of 17% from the flour enriched at 1 μg/g and of 8% from that enriched at 5 μg/g.

Similarly, 11% of added pteroylglutamic acid was lost on baking into bread while 30% of the vitamin naturally present was destroyed. The authors showed that this baking loss was compensated by the gain in folate during fermentation of the dough – there was a 65% increase in total folic acid synthesised by the yeast so that there was no aggregate loss during baking.

Section C

Effects of Processes

Chapter 7

Foods are subjected to a vast number of processes – blanching, pasteurisation, sterilisation, dehydration, freezing, fermenting, cooking – all of which cause some change in nutritional values.

The greatest loss of nutrients, which is discussed under several headings, is by extraction into water and by heat damage. Thermal degradation of nutrients has been extensively studied in attempts to arrive at methods of predicting losses; kinetic data on this subject were reviewed by Lund (1975) [525].

The activation energy required for the destruction of some of the more heat-resistant enzymes is comparable with that which damages some of the nutrients, and the activation energy required to destroy spores of microorganisms can be greater. For a given increase in temperature the rate of destruction of microorganisms (a biological effect) increases faster than nutrient destruction (a chemical reaction) and investigation of these conditions points to optimum processing conditions, i.e. least damage to nutrients and other food qualities. However, as Lund (1975) [525] concluded, the data available for prediction are inadequate in most, if not all, instances.

Conditions for maximum nutrient retention are not always the same as those conferring maximum palatability. Food may be completely cooked when measured by the criterion of texture, i.e. cell walls may be sufficiently softened, but maximum palatability might not be achieved without additional cooking, with possible further destruction of nutrients. For example, roasting and toasting confer a desirable flavour accompanied by loss of nutritional value. Considerable differences between adequate and desirable cooking might exist with foods like legumes which, in the laboratory, can be cooked until they are soft while traditional cooking may continue for many hours longer to produce the desired flavour. Such prolonged cooking is likely to affect the quality of the proteins but does not appear to have been investigated.

DEVELOPMENTS IN PROCESSING METHODS

Advances in food technology can lead to differences in nutritive value in the newer product which may be higher or lower than the more traditional product. Some methods, designed to retain as much as possible of the

95

original flavour, colour and texture of the food are less severe than those they replace, such as vacuum and freeze-drying and ultra-high temperature sterilisation, and therefore tend to result in smaller losses of nutrients. Other changes such as from free-range to broiler chickens, manufacture of bread by the Continuous-Dough-Mix or Chorleywood Process, or the intensive rearing of beef might affect nutrients in either direction, particularly as they often involve new strains of plants and animals.

Tolan *et al.* (1974) studied the chemical composition of eggs from hens reared under the (older) free range, deep litter and (modern) battery conditions. There was no difference in protein, fats (cholesterol, tri-glycerides, phospholipids, essential fatty acids), and most vitamins (thiamin, riboflavin, niacin, pantothenic acid, vitamin A). The only differences were that battery hens produced eggs with 10% more calcium, 40% less folic acid and 30% less vitamin B_{12}; deep litter eggs had 20% more vitamin E. However, variations in the compositions of eggs from different farms were greater than those caused by the system of management [511].

As discussed under Cereals (p. 139) the Continuous-Dough-Mix and the Chorleywood methods of bread-making have no material effect on nutritional value compared with conventional methods [232, 263].

Other new processes include the change from free-range to broiler chickens [83] and from extensive to intensive rearing of beef [37]. These were not significantly different from the older products but, on the other hand, dehydrated potatoes are considerably poorer than whole potatoes in vitamin C and thiamin unless they have been enriched.

Mechanical harvesting can be included among newer methods. This has long been used for foods such as potatoes, carrots and peas but has been applied to cherries and tomatoes relatively recently. The main effect of interest is the bruising involved which can break down cell structure and, so far as nutrition is concerned, this would damage the vitamin C. If tomatoes are harvested mechanically this is usually done while they are still green and the cell walls are strong enough to withstand the bruising; consequently they are finally matured off the vine with a reduction of about 30% of the vitamin C compared with harvesting when ripe [371].

PASTEURISATION AND STERILISATION

These are amongst the commonest methods of preserving foods of all types. Sterilisation lengthens shelf life indefinitely but the relatively severe treatment usually required spoils texture, colour, flavour and nutritional value. Pasteurisation is less severe and does less damage but, even when used in conjunction with other methods such as cooling and irradiation, has only a limited effect on shelf life. Since increasing the temperature of treatment has a greater effect on microorganisms than on nutrients much effort has been devoted to processes such as High-temperature-short-time and Ultra-high-temperature treatments [653, 525].

BLANCHING

Blanching is an essential preliminary before freezing, drying and canning and consists of subjecting the food to a high temperature for a few minutes. This serves to inactivate the enzymes which would otherwise cause deterioration during storage of frozen foods, to wilt bulky vegetables and reduce their volume prior to canning, to expel gases that might create excessive pressure in the can and to maintain colour; at the same time, blanching serves as a cleaning process.

One of the commonest methods is immersion in hot water but a variety of other methods including hot air, steam and irradiation are in use. This topic has been extensively reviewed by Lund (1975) [525] and Fennema (1975) [581]. The time of treatment varies with the food, its size and the particular process used, e.g. it may vary from 3.5 min for small Brussels sprouts to 7 min for the largest size; garden peas are satisfactorily treated in 1 min, sliced beans may require 2 min, and temperatures range from 93 to 99°C [514].

In the blanching and subsequent water-cooling losses of soluble nutrients such as mineral salts, small amounts of protein, sugars and vitamins, are inevitable and will vary with the size of the piece of food, the product-to-water ratio, degree of stirring of the blanching water, temperature and concentration of solids in the water. Oxidation also occurs [315].

Adam et al. (1942) [513] found that half the vitamin C could be lost in 6 min from vegetables with a large surface – area-to-volume ratio such as peas, sliced beans and sliced and diced carrots. Vegetables with a smaller surface – area-to-volume such as whole beans, potatoes and sprouts lost one third of the vitamin C. These authors found little difference with times between 1 and 6 min. They also showed a differential loss between sugars and minerals which may be due, as Birch et al. (1974) [315] showed for peas, to the fact that the concentration of the nutrients is not uniform in the foodstuff. For example, the concentration of vitamin C is greater in the testa of the pea so that the rate of extraction into the water is greater in the early stages and the loss of the vitamin therefore does not parallel the loss of other solids and is not proportional to time of treatment.

The loss of vitamin C is effected by extraction and enzymic destruction. Birch et al. (1974) [315] found that treatment at 85°C inactivated the enzymes and so the extracted vitamin C was recovered completely in the blanching water. At the lower temperature of 70°C the enzymes were not inactivated and there was enzymic destruction of the vitamin as well as extraction – 24% was oxidised in 2 min.

There is a great variation from one factory to another because of the different equipment, times and temperatures employed; the degree of maturity of the vegetables may also have an effect. Cameron *et al.* (1949) [552] compared results from different factories and found very large differences both in leafy and solid vegetables: per cent losses were:

	Vitamin C	Niacin	Riboflavin	Thiamin
Asparagus	0–15	0–23	0–18	0–20
Green beans	10–50	0–40	0–30	0–20
Peas	10–30	5–40	13–33	0–37
Spinach	0–95	0–37	0–22	0–33

The addition of 2% sodium chloride to the blanching water has been claimed to reduce the loss of vitamin C but Hudson, Sharple *et al.* (1974) on a domestic scale found that the addition of 1.2% sodium chloride or sucrose had no effect on the number of vegetables [522].

Steam blanching involves less water but a longer time may be needed to inactivate the enzymes compared with boiling water so while less material may be extracted oxidation may be occurring (513 370). At the same time the colour may be adversely affected but the inclusion of ammonia with the steam maintains a higher pH and stabilises the chlorophyll [370].

In general losses appear to be less with steam blanching although some workers failed to find any difference, possibly because effects vary with the type of food [456]. See Table 7.1.

The considerable losses of folic acid that occur in canning are mainly at the blanching stage. Lin *et al.* (1975) [440] showed that only 5% of the folate of Garbanzo beans was lost in a 12 h preliminary soaking, and 10% during sterilisation but major losses occurred during blanching. Steam was superior to water; in water at 100°C losses were 20%, 25% and 45% in 5, 10 and 20 min respectively; corresponding losses in steam were half these, namely 10%, 20% and 25%.

Microwave blanching is reported to cause less damage than steam, and a combination of methods such as microwave treatment and hot water has been claimed to achieve a better product from the point of view of palatability and nutritional value, but this can depend on the product in question [515].

In fluidised-bed blanching of peas less is extracted than by wet methods [528]. In spinach less carotene was damaged with the hot-gas process – the treated material contained 5.4 mg carotene per 100 g compared with 3.9

after water treatment [531]. Similarly vitamin C was better retained – 34 mg per 100 g after gas treatment compared with 21 mg after water treatment.

Lund (1975) [525] summarised the literature as follows: loss of vitamin C:—asparagus, 10%, green beans, Lima beans, sprouts, cauliflower and peas, 20–25%, broccoli 35%, spinach 50%. Loss of thiamin:—peas and green beans 10%, Lima beans 35% and spinach 60%. Carotene is generally stable.

TABLE 7.1. Losses of vitamin C during blanching

Food	Method	Temp. (°C)	Time (min)	Loss (%)	Reference
Broccoli	Water	100	3	30	Eheart (1970) [516]
				40	Noble *et al.* (1964) [530]
			4	50	Odland *et al.* (1975) [370]
		77	10	30	Eheart (1970)
	Steam		4	20	Odland *et al.* (1975)
			6	40	Noble *et al.* (1964)
	Steam-NH₃		6	40	Odland *et al* (1975)
	Microwave		2	20	Eheart (1970)
Sprouts	Water	100	3	25	Noble *et al.* (1964)
			3.5	15	
			4.5	15	Abrams (1975) [308]
			5.5	20	
	Steam		4	15	Noble *et al.* (1964)

Since the overall losses involved in both canning and drying are incurred largely at the blanching stage there is little overall difference between these two methods of processing (Tables 1.1 and 1.2, chapter 1).

In the preparation of certain dietetic foods it is important to note that blanching water can increase the calcium and sodium content of the food.

DRYING

Proteins

Where heat is the main cause of damage the drying process usually has little effect on protein quality unless the temperature of the food is allowed to rise above 100°C. So long as there is free escape of steam the temperature of the heated food cannot rise above 100°C while moisture is present, however rapid the heat input. Thus it has been reported that even flame drying of fish meal with incoming air as hot as 1100°C did not damage the protein quality of the bulk of the product, only that of the material crusted onto the sides of the dryer. Once the material has dried its temperature will, of course, rapidly rise to that of the heating surface. The interior of a loaf of bread does not rise above 95°C in an oven at 300°C but that of the crust does rise above this temperature. The protein inside the loaf is little damaged, but the available lysine content of the crust is reduced.

TABLE 7.2. Protein quality – Cooked vs cooked and dehydrated foods (De Groot, 1963) [533]

	Biological value		Digestibility	
	Cooked	Dried	Cooked	Dried
Cabbage (1)	0.40	0.35	0.88	0.89
Lima beans (2)	0.58	0.56	0.87	0.87
Red beans (3)	0.45	0.49	0.78	0.75
Green beans (4)	0.57	A 0.57	0.82	A 0.81
		B 0.59		B 0.80
		C 0.54		C 0.81
		D 0.52		D 0.72
Turnip greens (5)	0.52	0.53	0.86	0.86
Kale (6)	0.64	0.61	0.85	0.85
Sweet corn (7)	0.76	0.75	0.97	0.98
Fish (haddock, boiled) (8)	0.83	0.84	1.00	1.00
Fish patties (raw mixture BV 0.87) (9)	0.83	0.84	0.98	0.99
Egg preparation (10)	0.94	E 0.94	0.98	E 0.98
		F 0.93		F 0.97
Beef, boiled (11)	0.74	0.74	1.00	1.00
Chicken, boiled (12)	0.72	0.74	1.00	1.00
Cheese (13)	0.70	0.70	0.99	0.99

Dehydration conditions
(1) 71°C for 2 h, then 49°C for 0.5 h.
(2), (3) 71°C for 4 h, then 49″C for 12 h.
(4) A: 71°C for 0.5 h, then 60°C for 1 h and 49°C for 20 h, B: vacuum
    dried, C: freeze-dried, D: *canned* 116°C for 35 min.
(5), (6) 63°C for 4 h, then 49°C for 12 h.
(7), (8), (11), (12), (13) Freeze-dried.
(9) Fried 200°C for 2.5 min, then freeze-dried.
(10) Egg, milk powder, cottonseed oil: E: pasteurised, F: spray-dried.

Lower temperatures can damage proteins in the presence of reducing substances and Duckworth and Woodham (1961) found a decrease in the protein quality of leaf extracts when the temperature of the material reached 82°C [323].

De Groot (1963) [533] examined protein quality (both digestibility and BV) on 12 cooked foods and showed no change on drying (at least as regards the limiting amino acids). See Table 7.2.

Cabbage was dried after cooking and sulphiting by a stream of air at 71°C for 2 h and 49°C for another 0.5 h. There was an apparent small, but not statistically significant fall from BV 0.40 to 0.35: digestibility was unchanged.

Lima beans and red beans dried for 4 h at 71°C and left 12 h at 49°C showed no loss. Green beans dried in hot air, and freeze-dried showed no change. Similar turnip greens and kale dried 4 h at 63°C and overnight at 49°C, freeze-dried sweet corn, freeze-dried fish, beef and chicken, freeze-dried fish patties, freeze-dried cheese and spray-dried pasteurised egg were all stable with regards to digestibility and BV of the proteins.

After drying subsequent loss of protein quality during cool storage is slow, so long as moisture is kept below about 5%. The protein quality of corn-soy-milk mixture was unchanges on storage at −18°C for one year. At 25°C the loss was 20% and at 48°C was 75% [885].

Wheat flour stored in airtight bags at 38°C retained 90% of the nutritive value after 6 months; in sealed jars it showed the same stability for 12 months. Parallel figures were collected for skim dried milk powder – higher storage temperatures were permitted at 40% relative humidity than at 60%. There was, however, still a slow loss in terms of PER when sealed in vacuum unless the temperature was maintained at −15°C.

Vitamins

As in almost all methods of processing vitamin C is the most unstable nutrient. Equipment that leads to shorter drying times therefore improves its retention. In vacuum puff-drying of tomato juice concentrate there was virtually no loss of vitamin C despite the aeration that is needed for the puffing [538a].

The storage of the dried food can result in losses. Kramer (1974) [902] and Bluestein and Labuza (1975) [532] reviewed the literature and the former summarised maximum temperatures and moisture levels which would allow full retention of the vitamins. For example, at 1.5% moisture and 4°C there was no loss of vitamin C from dried tomato flakes after one year. At 1% moisture at 21°C 10% was lost, and this loss increased to 30% at 5% moisture.

CANNING

Although canned foods, being sterile, have an indefinite life from the microbiological point of view, there is a decline in organoleptic and nutritional properties during storage due to chemical reactions [553, 560]. Bender (1966) [883] examined the NPU of two samples of meat (veal and mutton) that had been canned 110 and 136 years earlier respectively. The contents were still sterile but NPU had fallen to 0.29 and 0.37 respectively. Acid hydrolysis revealed that all the amino acids were present to the same extent as in fresh meat so it would appear that this loss was due to the amino acids becoming unavailable through chemical change.

There are several changes that can occur in canned foods. First, there can be destruction of nutrients during the sterilisation process. Secondly, there is inevitably a leaching of water-soluble nutrients from the food into the liquor – this is a loss only if the liquor is discarded. Thirdly, there can be a slow chemical destruction during storage depending on a variety of factors such as temperature, residual oxygen and the metallic surface of the container. An example of the last is the greater loss of vitamin C that takes place in lacquered cans compared with plain ones; in unlacquered cans the residual oxygen is rapidly used up in the electrochemical process of corrosion – at least with acidic foods [308]. In fact this often leads to better retention of vitamin C in fruit products packed in plain tin cans than in glass bottles.

Losses during processing and subsequent storage are exemplified by the findings of Hellendoorn et al. (1971) [560]..A mixture of spinach, pork and potatoes had NPU 0.68 before canning, which fell to 0.60 after canning, to 0.57 after 3 years storage and to 0.55 after 5 years. Another product, goulash with potatoes, showed no change on sterilising but NPU fell from 0.64 to 0.55 after 3 years and 0.52 after 5 years storage (see under Meat, p. 123).

De Groot (1963) examined protein quality of green beans after cooking and sulphiting. The canning process reduced BV from 0.57 to 0.52 and digestibility from 0.82 to 0.72 (i.e. NPU from 0.46 to 0.38) [533].

Hellendoorn et al. (1971) [560] found that most of the vitamins were stable both to processing and storage at 22°C with the exception of vitamin A and thiamin, which were originally present in only small quantities (Table 7.3). Half of the vitamin A was destroyed during processing and the remainder was lost after 1.5 years storage. Half of the thiamin was destroyed during processing and the loss increased to 75% after 1.5 years.

Pantothenate was relatively unstable, 25% being lost during processing and 50% after 1.5 years. Niacin was the only other vitamin to suffer any loss and this was only 10% through processing, increasing to 20% after 1.5 years storage. Vitamins B_2, B_6, B_{12}, folate, inositol and choline were stable; vitamin E was stable to processing but half was lost during 3 years storage.

The values shown in Table 7.3 are the average of six types of food which differed to some extent in their behaviour. For example, there was no loss of vitamin A in two of the foods, Dun peas with bacon, and white beans with bacon, potatoes and tomato sauce.

Cameron (1955) [550] had also shown that the major changes take place

TABLE 7.3. Vitamin losses after canning and storage of whole meals (22±2°C) (per cent loss) (from Hellendoorn *et al.*, 1971 [560])

Vitamin	Initial value	After canning	1.5 years	Storage 3 years	5 years
Vitamin A	16.5 μg	50	100	—	—
Vitamin E	80 mg	0	0	50	50
Thiamin	9 mg	50	75	75	75
Riboflavin	6 mg	0	0	0	0
Pyridoxine	5 mg	0	0	0	0
Vitamin B_{12}	18 μg	0	0	0	0
Niacin	110 mg	10	20	20	20
Pantothenate	21 mg	25	50	50	50
Folic acid	14 μg	0	0	0	0
Inositol	26 mg	0	0	0	0
Choline	27 mg	0	0	0	0

TABLE 7.4. Vitamin losses during storage in cans (per cent loss)

Food	Temp. (°C)	Vitamin	1 year	2 years	Ref.
Peas	10–27	C	10	10	1
		B_1	10–15	10–20	1
		Carotene	0–5	5–10	1
Orange juice	10–27	C	5–20	20–40	1
	10;18		0		2
	27		25		2
	10–27	B_1	0	10–20	1
	10;18		0		2
	27		10		2
	10–27	Carotene	0	0–20	1
Tomato juice	10–27	C	0–20	0–20	1
	10;18		0		2
	27		25		
	10–27	B_1	5–10	10–30	1
	27		10		2
Grapefruit juice	10;18	C	0		2
	27	C	25		2
	27	B_1	10		2
Pineapple juice	10;18	C	0		2
	27	C	10		2
	27	B_1	10		2

[1] Monroe *et al.*, 1949 [567]; Sheft *et al.*, 1949 [569]; Guerrant *et al.*, 1948 [558].
[2] Cameron, 1955 [550].

during the sterilising process itself and subsequent losses during storage are slow. The following range of losses from tomato juice took place during canning: vitamin C 10–65%, thiamin 0–27%, riboflavin 0–14%, niacin 0–17%, carotene 25–40%. During storage there was no loss at 10°C and 18°C, only at 27°C. Table 7.4 shows these results together with a series of measurements made on canned peas, tomatoes and orange juice that had been stored under commercial conditions in a number of warehouses for 1 and 2 years at temperatures averaging between 10 and 27°C [557, 567, 569].

Kramer (1974) [902] reviewed the literature and concluded that canned fruit juices lost insignificant amounts of vitamin C after one year storage at 4°C. At 27°C the loss was 25% after 1 year and 50% after 2 years. Carotene was more stable and there was no loss from carrot juice stored at ambient temperature for one year.

TABLE 7.5. Range of values found in samples of canned foods (mg/100 g food) (Tepley et al., 1953 [571])

	Mean	Range	No. samples
Vitamin B$_6$			
Apple juice	0.035	3½-fold	4
Asparagus	0.075	5	7
Green beans	0.043	8	10
Pineapple juice	0.33	2½	5
Tuna fish	0.67	2	4
β-Carotene			
Cranberry sauce	0.009	50-fold	7
Pumpkin	6.8	12	5
Sweet potatoes	3.8	3	6
Thiamin, riboflavin and niacin			
Chicken: thiamin	0.003	2-fold	6
riboflavin	0.1	2	3
niacin	5.5	2	3
Chili con carné: thiamin	0.032	2½	5
riboflavin	0.083	1½	5
niacin	1.6	2	5
Clams: thiamin	0.009	10	5
riboflavin	0.09	3	5
niacin	1.0	7	5
Oysters: thiamin	0.02	3	3
riboflavin	0.2	3	3
niacin	1	3	3
Tuna fish: thiamin	0.02	3½	4
riboflavin	0.09	2	4
niacin	14	1½	4

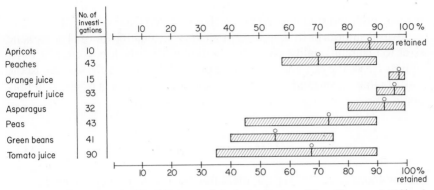

FIG. 7.1. Vitamin C retained in canned fruits and vegetables. Range of 90% of findings, 0 indicated median value. (After Zacharias, 1965 [737])

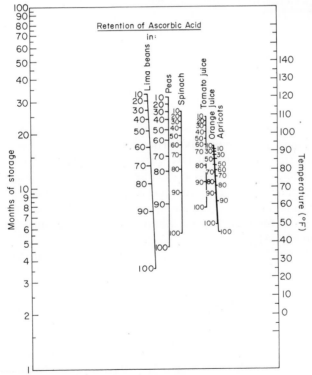

FIG. 7.2. Proposed nomograph for the stability of ascorbic acid in canned foods. (Freed *et al.*, 1949 [556])

Figure 7.1 shows the range of vitamin C retention reported by a series of investigators and summarised by Zacharias (1965) [737] see also Table 7.5.

Several authors have suggested methods of evaluating thermal processing so as to maintain quality while effectively sterilising the food [554, 653, 631]. Others ([556, Fig. 7.2 and [735]) have proposed nomographs to forecast the loss of vitamins in canned foods during storage but these are not generally applicable.

Metal contamination

Hellendoorn *et al.* (1971) [560] measured the uptake of metal from the cans during storage and found that this varied with the product; Dun peas with bacon contained only 2 ppm of tin after 5 years, while beans, bacon and potatoes, the most acid product, contained 38 ppm. The contamination took place after sterilisation during storage.

The amount of lead was small, finishing at 0.4 ppm while the initial values were stated as being less than 0.2 ppm. Figures given for iron indicated no pick-up.

FREEZING

Both from the organoleptic and nutritional points of view freezing is the best method of preserving food. The temperature of storage must be a compromise between optimal and practical and is usually −18°C. There is still a slow deterioration of food qualities but this is acceptable. Losses of nutrients depend on temperature; for example, there is a slow loss of vitamin C in most foods at −18°C compared with losses two to five times as fast at −10°C (except for orange juice where losses are the same at these two temperatures) [581].

Even at −30°C part of the water is still unfrozen and slow chemical deterioration takes place. The concentration of cell materials can cause local changes in pH leading to destruction of some of the nutrients, particularly vitamin C and, as described earlier, the relative stability of lipid hydroperoxides at low temperatures leads to loss of vitamin E during frozen storage.

The principal loss of nutrients in this process does not occur during the freezing itself but in the preliminary blanching that is necessary to destroy the enzymes as already discussed. There are no losses during the freezing operation, except for vitamin C and even these are only 0–10% [581]. A second opportunity for loss occurs during thawing which is carried out in the home under a variety of uncontrolled conditions and can lead to changes of osmotic pressure within the tissues of the thawing food with some, usually small, destruction of nutrients and also of textural properties.

Frozen vs 'fresh'

The literature reveals considerable variations in the stability of nutrients in frozen foods which may be partly due to different processing conditions but also because of the varying extent of inactivation of oxidising enzymes in the blanching process. Furthermore, there is evidence that reactivation of enzymes can occur.

The nutritive value of frozen foods can be higher or lower than that of the fresh food, higher because foods are frozen immediately after harvesting, lower because of losses in blanching. Fresh foods, better termed 'market fresh', may have been stored at ambient temperatures for several days with some loss of nutrients (mostly vitamin C); foods are mostly at their peak of nutrient content at the time of harvesting.

A complicating factor is that while blanching removes some nutrients it preserves the remainder by destroying oxidising enzymes. Finally, errors have arisen in interpretation through comparing frozen foods (after thawing) with fresh samples without taking into account the fact that the latter would require longer cooking. The proper comparison must be the final cooked foods on the plate. For example as shown earlier (Tables 1.1 and 1.2) it is clear that there is little difference after final cooking between the vitamin C contents of fresh peas and those processed by freezing or freeze-drying.

A useful series of comparable figures for losses of vitamins was given by Weits *et al.* (1970) [390]. Spinach lost 60% of its vitamin C on blanching and freezing, which was the same as the loss in freshly cooked foods. There was an additional loss of 10% during 6 months storage and a final loss of 10% (i.e. 80% in all) in the final cooking.

Peas lost 40% during blanching and freezing but there was no loss during 6 months storage; the final cooking caused an additional loss of 30%.

French beans lost less – 25% – during blanching and freezing, nil during storage, 25% on final cooking – total 50%.

Losses of thiamin from spinach were considerable at the first stage – 80% compared with only 40% on cooking of the fresh food. There was no loss on storage (final cooking loss was not given). Thiamin in French beans, however, was more stable – only 10% loss on blanching and freezing, the same as when cooked fresh, with no further loss on storage and final cooking.

Riboflavin losses from peas were 40% on blanching compared with 20%

fresh-cooked; an additional loss of 5% took place during storage and another 5% on final cooking, totalling 50%.

Some typical losses of vitamin C were given by Clegg (1974) [577] – cumulative percentage losses on a wet weight basis:

	Peas	Sliced beans	Sprouts
Since harvesting	5	4	1
Blanching	20	12	32*
Cooling	20	20	32*
Freezing	20	24	30*

* The considerable losses from the sprouts were largely due to the increased water content — on a dry weight basis the loss was only 10%.

A large number of frozen foods totalling 27 000 packages from 150 freezing plants were examined for 8 vitamins and 6 minerals in the 1953 and 1954 production seasons [318] and the results give some idea of the natural plus processing variations. For 20 samples of spinach the range of vitamin C content was 8–45 mg/100 g; for 28 samples of sprouts 70–105 mg. For carotene the range was 0.8–2.7 mg in 15 samples of broccoli and 0.03–0.13 mg/100 g in 15 samples of peas.

Niacin ranged between 0.9 and 1.7 mg in 32 samples of Lima beans; thiamin ranged between 0.12 and 0.23 in 18 samples of asparagus.

Such a range of vitamin concentration is well recognised, but there was also a variation, although smaller, in protein content. In 18 samples of asparagus spears protein varied between 2.7 and 3.9%; in 23 samples of French beans, 1.3 and 2.0%; and in 15 samples of chopped broccoli, 2.5 and 4.4%. A small amount of protein may have been extracted during blanching, the remainder of the variation is due to the raw material.

Possibly the greatest range of variation, although a matter of specialised interest, was from 0.9 to 12.8 mg sodium per 100 g in only 8 samples of rhubarb.

Fennema (1975) concluded from a review of the literature that vitamin C and pantothenate are the most labile nutrients during frozen storage, thiamin being slightly more stable [581].

Kramer (1974) attempted to relate the retention of vitamin C to general quality changes during storage but some foods lost as much as 50% of their vitamin C in one year at −5°C while still maintaining sensory qualities [902].

Animal products

The only pre-treatment in freezing meat is aging, just as for fresh meat. Meyer *et al.* (1963) found 35% loss of niacin but no loss of thiamin or riboflavin from meat held at 1°C for 21 days [61]; Fennema (1975) concluded that short-term aging has little or no effect [581].

Freezing has no effect on B vitamins but the rate of freezing can influence the subsequent losses of exudate during thawing and cooking. During frozen storage the thiamin, riboflavin, niacin and pantothenate, appear, from the limited amount of information available, to be stable while there are losses of pyridoxine [49].

During thawing there is a loss in the juices of about 10% of the water-soluble B vitamins [92, 587]. Similar losses occur in thawing frozen fish [110]. Fennema (1975) summarised the literature findings of losses of B vitamins from meat and poultry during freezing and storage (excluding subsequent cooking); figures vary considerably from zero to 30% for thiamin, riboflavin, niacin and pyridoxine after 6–12 months at −18°C [581].

De Ritter *et al.* (1974) examined a number of frozen meals and found very wide ranges of vitamin losses in preparation and cooking – losses of vitamin C were between 50% and 100%. In some foods this was the only loss; in other foods up to 25% of B_6 and niacin, 33% of vitamin E, 55% of vitamin A and 85% of thiamin were lost [578].

Reheating

Even careful reheating at 70-80°C caused a loss of 20% of the ascorbic acid from frozen spinach and sprouts [580]. Since temperature is the critical factor the oven design, depth of packing the food and rate of heating govern the losses. Eddy *et al.* (1968) point out that the ideal pack would expose the maximum surface area to the heat source with the minimum practical depth [580].

Thawing, as mentioned earlier, can cause textural damage depending on the rate of thawing, which will involve the size of the sample of food and heat penetration. There is only a limited amount of evidence available about nutritional damage at this stage.

Hucker and Clarke (1961) thawed foods at low temperatures of 2, 7 and 21°C and refroze them through repeated cycles and concluded that at these temperatures time was the important factor. Moreover, foods varied in their susceptibility to nutritional damage – six cycles of thawing and refreezing extending over 3 h destroyed 50% of the vitamin C in maize but none of that of green beans, peas and Lima beans [585].

Some workers have concluded that different methods of reheating, such as microwave compared with conventional gas ovens did not make any difference [9, 575, 576] while others found less damage with microwave and infrared heating because of the shorter time required [574]. Bulk foods required frequent stirring to avoid scorching and this tended to oxidise the vitamin C. These authors emphasise that the results varied with the type of food.

The subject of reheating was reviewed by Lachance *et al.* (1973) [903].

The greatest losses of vitamin C and thiamin take place when food is kept hot and the cook-freeze-thaw system [887] is designed to overcome this by making food available for consumption soon after the final reheating. This method gave greater retention of vitamin C and a slight superiority in available lysine but no difference in thiamin and riboflavin. Head (1974) [896] examined food prepared in a central kitchen and transported to various schools; under those particular conditions vitamin C was partly oxidised but thiamin and riboflavin were stable. The B vitamins were shown to be stable in slices of meat kept hot [10, 29, 574].

PRESSURE COOKING

It is often assumed that pressure cooking has an advantage over boiling since the heating time is shorter and less of the soluble nutrients should be leached out. However, some of the reported results are conflicting and there are marked differences between the nutrients.

For example, Munsell *et al.* (1949) [366] showed smaller losses of vitamins from cabbage cooked under pressure than with boiling, namely, 33% loss of vitamin C compared with 70%, 12% loss of thiamin compared with 55%, and zero for riboflavin compared with 50%. The principal cause of loss is by leaching, rather than heat as illustrated by Krehl and Winters (1950) [354]. These authors compared the loss of four vitamins and two minerals from a variety of vegetables cooked: (*a*) under pressure with 125 ml water, (*b*) in an open pan with the minimum of water, (*c*) in an open pan with 125 ml of water. Portions were 'family size' and each food was cooked to the same degree of tenderness so that the time varied with the food and the method. With the same volume of water there was little difference between open pan and pressure cooking, despite the difference in times. The greatest loss occurred with the larger volumes of water and losses were least with 'waterless cooking' (Table 7.6). Similarly, Trefether *et al.* (1951) found virtually no difference between open pan boiling for 13 min, and pressure cooking at 5 lb for 7 min, 10 lb for 6 min and 15 lb for 5.5 min for ascorbic acid, thiamin and riboflavin [386].

Noble (1967) [367a] on the other hand showed a clear advantage for pressure cooking in retention of vitamin C in a variety of vegetables.

More recently Kamalanathan *et al.* (1972, 1974) [350] showed with several vegetables that pressure cooking with a loss of 25–50% of the thiamin, was better than steaming with 50% loss, and much better than boiling with

TABLE 7.6. Loss of nutrients from family size portions of food cooked by different methods. 1. pressure cooking (125 ml water), 2. pan cooking with minimum of water, 3. pan cooking with 125 ml water, 4. 'waterless cooking' (adapted from Krehl and Winters (1950) [354], figures rounded off.)

Cooking method		Calcium	Iron	Vitamin			
				B_1	B_2	Niacin	C
Asparagus	1	6	10	20	30	15	30
	2	12	20	45	40	40	60
	3	7	10	30	40	20	30
	4	0	3	10	20	10	30
Beets	1	5	6	20	10	10	5
	2	15	15	40	30	30	25
	3	10	10	30	15	15	10
	4	0	3	10	10	5	20
Broccoli	1	7	10	20	10	25	30
	2	16	15	30	35	55	50
	3	12	10	25	25	15	30
	4	4	5	5	20	5	30
Cabbage	1	9	10	30	15	25	25
	2	20	15	40	50	50	55
	3	12	5	30	30	30	40
	4	4	5	10	15	15	30
Carrots	1	10	15	15	10	10	20
	2	20	20	30	25	25	40
	3	10	10	15	15	10	25
	4	5	10	5	5	0	30
Cauliflower	1	10	20	25	25	25	25
	2	20	25	50	40	40	50
	3	15	20	30	25	25	55
	4	10	10	10	15	10	30
Corn	1	15	20	20	20	20	25
	2	20	30	30	50	50	40
	3	10	15	20	15	15	35
	4	10	10	10	10	10	30
Peas	1	15	20	20	20	10	25
	2	20	20	40	25	30	50
	3	15	15	20	10	20	30
	4	5	10	5	5	5	10
Potatoes	1	20	25	15	20	20	40
	2	45	40	30	35	35	60
	3	25	30	20	20	25	50
	4	10	15	10	10	10	20
Spinach	1	15	15	25	25	30	40
	2	25	20	50	45	60	50
	3	20	15	30	30	25	50
	4	10	10	10	15	10	30

75–80% loss. For vitamin C the results depended on the vegetable; amaranth leaves lost 80% under pressure, and 70% on steaming; French beans lost nothing when cooked in an open pan with the minimum of water, and 30% both on steaming and under pressure. Drumstick leaves lost 50%, 30% and 25% respectively by these three methods.

Consequently no general conclusions can be drawn about the relative value of pressure cooking as such, since so many factors from type of food to volumes of water must be taken into account.

IONISING RADIATION

This refers to cathode rays, X-rays and gamma rays used to destroy microorganisms, inhibit sprouting of potatoes, disinfest wheat and extend the shelf-life of fish and poultry. Gamma radiation is the form most frequently used.

Doses sufficiently high to sterilise foods (5-6 Mrad-radappertisation) produce strong off-flavours, especially in fish and meat, so lower doses of about 0.2 to 1.0 Mrad are mostly used to pasteurise (radicidation) sometimes in conjunction with mild heat treatment. At such levels the effects on nutrients are similar to those of other methods of processing. (Reviewed by Reber *et al.*, 1966 and Josephson *et al.*, 1975 [646, 620].)

Proteins

Proteins are little affected by doses in the range 0.2–1.0 Mrad. Disinfestation of wheat flour with 0.2 Mrad had no effect on the BV [650]. Nor was there any fall in the BV of fish treated with 0.6–1.0 Mrad although there was some damage to the cysteine [120, 657].

Some of the reports are conflicting but it appears that the higher doses that cause off-flavours do affect proteins slightly; 1.5 Mrad causes destruction of 5–10% of several of the amino acids. Methionine and histidine were the most sensitive, lysine being little damaged – only 6–8% destroyed even at 50 Mrad [630]; heterocyclic amino acids were damaged at 3 Mrad.

It is possible to reduce the cooking time of red gram by previously treating with 1 Mrad gamma radiation, with a parallel improvement of texture and without damage to the amino acids [449].

Some foods exhibit increased susceptibility to enzymic digestion, possibly due to partial protein breakdown or to the destruction of a trypsin inhibitor [449, 658, 271].

Potato proteins are affected; even the small doses used to inhibit the sprouting of potatoes – about 8 Krad – reduces BV from 0.80 to 0.73 after irradiation and 60 days storage. After 205 days the BV of control and treated samples were the same, namely 62 [660].

Some workers have reported that even at the high dose levels that give rise to off-flavours, protein damage is no greater than in heat processing. Johnson and Metta (1956) [271] found a fall in BV of 8% in milk irradiated with 3 Mrad, the same as after heat treatment; BV of beef was unchanged. Sheffner *et al.* (1957) [648] treated turkey with 2 Mrad and concluded that this gave a superior product to canned turkey, and that evaporated milk sterilised with this dose was similar to heat treated samples.

Vitamins

Thiamin is the most labile of the B vitamins; irradiation of fish with 0.6 Mrad destroyed 47% of the thiamin, only 6% of the riboflavin and none of the niacin; after subsequent cooking there was an additional loss of 10% of the riboflavin and the thiamin [120].

The stability of thiamin appears to vary with the food. Egg powder and maize lost none after treatment with 0.5 Mrad [612] while figs lost 40% when treated with a similar dose, 0.6 Mrad, for disinfestation [613a]. A smaller dose of 0.2 Mrad destroyed 10% of the thiamin, riboflavin and niacin of wheat [658] and 1 Mrad destroyed 10% of the natural thiamin and 20% of thiamin added to rice [612].

Pantothenate and pyridoxine in the rice were stable but pyridoxine is not always stable to irradiation since it can be lost from fish [657].

Reports of the stability of vitamin C are contradictory. There was no loss from bananas nor from potatoes treated with 8–10 Krad to prevent sprouting and stored 7 months [606a] but Gounelle *et al.* (1970) [612] reported loss of vitamin C during storage from both potatoes and carrots after irradiation and Proctor and Goldblith (1949) [614] reported earlier that ascorbic acid was the most sensitive of the vitamins. Milk irradiated with 440 Krad lost 40% of the carotenoids, 70% of the retinol and 60% of the tocopherol [623]. Vitamins in solution are usually far less stable than in foods.

In general, the nutritional effects of irradiation are similar to those of heat treatment; losses are minimised in the absence of oxygen and at low temperatures, and irradiation offers the advantage that it can be effectively carried out in frozen foods.

MICROWAVE HEATING

Microwave heating with high energy electromagnetic radiation (usually of frequency 2450 MHz, wavelength 12 cm) is an extremely efficient process entailing virtually no loss of energy compared with conventional cooking. In conventional cooking heat is applied to the surface of the food and then conducted to the inner parts with uneven distribution and possibly differential damage to the nutrients. Microwaves generate heat throughout the bulk of the food resulting in a more even temperature rise when the food is homogenous, but otherwise with 'hot spots'.

The method is very rapid and so is useful in flow systems, and it allows quick preparation of small quantities of food as required instead of keeping a large amount of food hot for long periods with detriment to palatability and nutrient content. It is also used to 'finish drying' potato chips and for cooking chicken pieces which are said to be juicier and more tender by this method.

Losses of nutrients are expected to be relatively low because of the lower surface temperature, the shorter time, and the low energy input, in-adequate, generally, to break chemical bonding. Reports of nutrient losses compared with conventional cooking, however, are not consistent. For example, there are reports of reduced losses of B vitamins from meat products and of vitamin C from vegetables conflicting with other reports where the authors failed to show any difference.

Campbell et al. (1958) [601] found only 10% loss of vitamin C from cabbage cooked 4 min by microwaves, compared with 50% in 3 min pressure cooking and 75% in conventional cooking. With fresh broccoli there was a loss of 40% in 3 min electronic cooking, almost as much as the 50% lost in 10 min conventional cooking. With frozen broccoli there was no loss in microwave cooking compared with 20% by conventional cooking. In these examples the change was measured in the food, no account being taken of the vitamins present in the cooking water.

Gordon and Noble (1959) [611] found microwave cooking superior to both boiling and pressure cooking, while Kylen et al. (1961) [624] and many other authors found no difference. The reasons for the apparent contradictions may lie in the findings of Ang and Livingstone (1974) [311] that the relative benefits of microwave cooking in respect of several of the vitamins vary with the food in question, apart from other differences in experimental conditions.

This suggestion is supported by the findings of Baldwin et al. (1976) [2] on cooking several types of meat at two 2450 MHz microwave ranges, viz. 220 and 115 volts, and in a conventional oven at 163°C. Less thiamin was lost from beef, pork and ham roasted in the microwave oven at 115 volts than by the other two methods. The different types of meat did not behave the same in all respects and the superiority of the microwave oven at 115 volts applied to riboflavin and niacin in beef and to niacin in pork. Thiamin losses in pork were lower than those reported by other workers.

Blanching by microwave treatment has an advantage over hot water since enzymes are more rapidly inactivated [593], but this does not necessarily run parallel with better retention of nutrients. Eheart (1967) [516] found a smaller loss of vitamin C (20%) from broccoli blanched electronically compared with water (40%) but greater destruction of chlorophyll during storage. In many instances the deterioration of colour and flavour would out-weigh the nutritional advantages.

Some of the problems involved in attempting to reach a conclusion are illustrated by the work of Wing and Alexander (1972) [663]. Chicken was cooked in only 1.5 min by microwave heating with an internal temperature of 96°C, compared with 45 min roasting with an internal temperature of 88°C. The authors concluded that microwave cooking destroyed significantly less vitamin B_6 but the difference was small, possibly within the error of measurement of this vitamin, and losses were largely recovered in the drippings. Microwave cooking caused a loss of 9% from the meat with 1.5% in the drippings, total loss 7.5%; roasting caused a loss of 17% with 5.4% in the drippings, total loss 11.6%. Since Miller et al. (1973) [445] found the coefficient of variation of analysis of vitamin B_6 to be 9% these figures do not indicate a real difference between the two methods.

Electronic cooking does not affect the fatty acids of meat [67].

FERMENTATION

It is traditional practice in the Far East to ferment cooked soybeans and cereal-legume mixtures with moulds or bacterial cultures. Natto or kojibean is a Japanese dish produced from soya by inoculation with *Bacillus natto*; miso is produced with *Aspergillus oryzae*; similar products such as tempeh are made in Indonesia.

Roelofsen and Talens (1964) [464] examined the changes in soya after fermentation with the mould *Rhizopus oryzae* and found a three-fold increase in riboflavin after 2 days and a six-fold increase after 3 days; niacin increased four-fold after 2 days. Thiamin fell by one-third since the mould requires this vitamin in the substrate. Murata et al. (1967) [447] found the same changes in tempeh, together with a marked increase in vitamin B_6 and pantothenate and a decrease in phytate [645].

It is not clear whether fermentation affects protein quality. A series of papers dealing with tempeh, natto, miso and tofu indicated no change but there were some inconsistencies [913a]. It was suggested that this might be partly explained by variations in the products; later workers [473] found no change on making tempeh while others reported a 15% fall in available lysine, which would not affect PER [658a]. Rajalakshmi and Vanaja (1967) [645] found an increase in PER from 1.5 to 2.0 in Idli (rice and black gram) and from 1.3 to 1.5 in khaman (Bengal gram). If the fermentation process merely made the product more palatable then the increased food intake would lead to a rise in PER so the reported improvements require confirmation.

Maize, whole grain or husked, is fermented and cooked by a number of different processes to form kenkey, commonly eaten in many parts of Africa. Ofusu (1971) [277] examined kenkey made by four different traditional methods. In two of these (Ga and Fante kenkey) the whole grain is used and there was no loss of available lysine compared with the raw maize (2.1 mg/g) and 10% loss of niacin (from 26 to 23 μg/g). Methods using husked grain showed losses of half the lysine and two-thirds of the niacin. A sample of Nsiho kenkey bought in the open market and made from husked grain had no detectable nitrogen!

OTHER METHODS
Micronisation

This is an extremely rapid method of heating with infrared radiation produced by heating propane on a ceramic tile or with nichrome wire elements [633]. It has been suggested as an alternative to steam heating or toasting where the shorter heating time might be less damaging e.g. 30–60 s at a temperature of 200–225°C. The biological value of soybeans was increased from its initial value of 0.53 to 0.73 [617] and vitamin E was not damaged [643].

Field beans so treated have an increased feed conversion efficiency when fed to animals, attributed partly to the destruction of trypsin inhibitors and partly to increased digestibility of the gelatinised starch. Available carbohydrate increased from 40% to 50% [633]. Similar improvements have been reported with micronisation of barley, wheat and maize when fed to pigs [626].

Intermediate moisture foods

Intermediate moisture foods containing 15–40% moisture lose available lysine during storage through Maillard reaction [627]. The fastest reaction is lipid oxidation resulting in rancid flavours, so limiting the shelf life of foods examined to a few weeks. Protection from oxidation makes non-enzymic browning the limiting reaction with respect to shelf life and since sugars are the most useful humectants there is little possibility of preventing this reaction by removing the sugars. There is rapid loss of nutrients especially vitamin C, which, at 25°C had a half-life of only 1 month unless the water content was reduced still further, but even then the shelf life was limited. At 45°C the half-life of vitamin C was only 1 day; thiamin was more stable with a half-life of 6 months at 25°C.

Chemical vs mechanical vs hand-peeling of vegetables

A range of vegetables (carrots, cucumber, parsley, kohl-rabi, potatoes and celery) were lye-peeled, peeled mechanically and by hand, and no difference was found in amounts of vitamin C and B_1 lost. Lye did not penetrate into the vegetables except for carrots, where the sodium level was increased [356].

Zarnegar and Bender (1971) attempted to ascertain whether the physical treatment incurred during mechanical peeling of potatoes was responsible for the loss of vitamin C and concluded that there was no such effect – the large losses reported in mechanical peeling appear to be caused by the prolonged soaking that it involves [500].

Gas storage

Fruits and vegetables can be stored by replacing the air first with carbon monoxide, which destroyes the enzymes, and then with ethylene oxide which destroys the microorganisms. Besser and Kramer (1972) [595] examined the effect of ethylene oxide on vitamin C since this gas is an oxidising agent. They found that peaches treated with carbon monoxide followed by nitrogen lost 50% of the vitamin C in 7 days at 3°C, with no further loss after 21 days. When the fruit was treated with carbon monoxide and ethylene oxide the loss of vitamin C was continuous and completed after 21 days.

These authors showed an apparent increase in thiamin in both mushrooms and minced beef patties on storage under nitrogen or carbon monoxide.

Pre-cooked and 'instantised' legumes

The long time and consequently considerable use of fuel needed to cook dried legumes has led to processing methods designed to reduce their cooking time. These consist of loosening the seed coats by either intermittent vacuum infiltration (Hydrovac process) or by blanching in steam or hot water or under pressure followed by soaking in a solution of various salts and finally drying to 6–7% moisture. These treated beans can be cooked in

10–15 min compared with five to six times as long for the unprocessed material. Trials on a variety of beans, peas and lentils showed that they had the same protein quality (measured by PER) as legumes cooked convention-ally [463]. Prolonged cooking both of processed and unprocessed legumes had some effect on lowering the protein quality.

Valledevi *et al.* (1972) [471] examined four pulses (Bengal gram, red gram, black gram and green gram) after cooking, drying and reconstituting in boiling water. Only black gram suffered severe losses, namely 40% of the thiamin, the others lost 15% thiamin, and the niacin and riboflavin were stable.

TABLE 7.7. Losses of vitamins in 'Instant bean powder' – pinto beans (per cent loss)
(Miller *et al.*, 1973 [445])

Nutrient	Treatment			
	A	B	C	D
Thiamin	20	20	60	70
Vitamin B_6	20	15	35	35
Niacin	20	0	40	50
Folate	20	60	40	40
PER	0.92	0.91	1.06	0.84

A. Cooked 1 h at 210°C, disintegrated and roller dried at 127°C 30 s.
B. Instantised by HCl treatment, pH 3.5, disintegrated, cooked, neutralised, dried.
C. Cooked 2 h, canned at 121°C 45 min.
D. Cooked 2 h, canned at 121°C 90 min.

Three months storage did not lead to any further loss from black gram but the other three samples lost 15–20% of the thiamin. There was no further loss after one year storage.

Pre-treatment with papain to tenderise the beans before dehydration had no additional effect.

Table 7.7 shows the losses from pinto beans precooked, 'instantised' and canned by two different processes compared with frozen beans used as controls. Except for thiamin the main loss was into the cooking water; the pre-cooked and 'instantised' products lost less thiamin, B_6 and niacin than the canned products but there was a large loss of folate on 'instantising' [445].

Extrusion cooking

This was originally evolved as a method of controlled heat destruction of toxins in soya meal required for poultry and pigfeed, and for gelatinisation of cereals. It is, effectively, high-temperature short-time heating and therefore likely to damage nutrients less than conventional heating. The process is commonly applied to enriched, high protein food preparations such as textured vegetable protein products and various mixtures based on soya that are designed as nutritional supplements, so retention of nutrients is a primary objective.

The foodstuff is subjected to gradually increasing temperature and pressure reaching 115 to 200°C for periods of 10–90 s. When it is finally extruded through a die or series of apertures the sudden reduction in pressure causes the superheated water to evaporate, the material expands and there is a laminar reorientation of the protein gel conferring a texture on the food, so long as starch is present. It is thus a highly appropriate method of converting powdered mixtures with nutrient additives into a texturised product.

TABLE 7.8. Effect of extrusion cooking on the nutritional value of soybeans (from Mustakas et al., 1970 [636])

Exit temp (°C)	135	121	135	135	149
Retention time (min)	1.25	2	1	2	1.25
Moisture (%)	15	20	25	20	20
PER	1.8	2.0	2.0	2.2	2.0
Available lysine					
% protein	6.1	6.3	6.3	6.3	6.2
Thiamin (mg/100 g)	0.85	0.85	0.75	0.82	0.74

Mustakas et al. (1964) examined the effects of a number of the variables on the nutritional value. There was no fall in NPU at what the authors termed low, medium and high temperature runs; NPU was 0.55 to 0.60 compared with 0.64 for a conventionally heated product but availably lysine ranged between 4.7 and 5.9%, indicating losses at some stage of the process [635].

Later, Mustakas et al. (1970) [636] gave the 'response contours' relating time of treatment to nutritional changes, flavour and stability (Table 7.8). PER increased up to the stage where 89% of the trypsin inhibitor had been inactivated and they concluded that to satisfy optimal peroxide value, flavour, urease activity and nutritional value the temperature should be within the range 121 to 138°C with a time–moisture range of 38–47. They showed that the process had little effect on thiamin, riboflavin and niacin while the conventionally-heated product lost 40% thiamin, no riboflavin and 60% of the niacin compared with the raw bean.

Muelenaere and Buzzard (1969) compared two cooker-extruder processes (the more complex Sprout-Waldron and the simpler Wenger) with conventional methods [634].

The processes include preconditioning with steam to a moisture content of

25% and heating to 93°C (when some degree of cooking is achieved) followed by 2–3 s heating at about 180°C in the extruder. Release of pressure leads to flash evaporation of some of the water, leaving about 18% moisture and forming an expanded product. These authors showed that the material was virtually sterilised in the process, trypsin inhibitor was 80–90% destroyed and the unpleasant flavours of the beans were removed.

In a corn-groundnut-soya mixture the following vitamin losses occurred:

Extrusion: 30% vitamin C, 3% niacin, 50% vitamin A.

Two min boiling (producing a similar product): 80% vitamin C, 6% niacin, 25% vitamin A.

As regards protein, measurement of available lysine showed that the Wenger process was less drastic than the Sprout-Waldron. A defatted soya-maize-sorghum mixture lost only 3% available lysine by the former process and 13% in the latter, compared with 20% on the roller dryer. Full fat soya showed no loss in the Wenger but there were no comparative figures for the other processes; a soy-milk-cereal preparation showed 28% loss in the Sprout-Waldron process.

Carnovale *et al.* (1969) reported that semolina or flour and water heated to 200°C for 30 min and extruded under pressure, as in the making of pasta, lost only 7% of the lysine and 7% of the threonine, but these were determined chemically so that there is no information of the loss of available amino acids [230].

Added amino acids were more labile: 25% of the lysine, 14% threonine and 18% of the methionine were destroyed.

Section D

Commodities

Chapter 8

MEAT AND MEAT PRODUCTS

In western diets meat is an important source of protein, iron and many B vitamins so it is the effect of processing on these nutrients that is of interest. The term 'meat' is popularly regarded as butcher's meat i.e. animal flesh; this contains a minimum of 10% fat, even when appearing to be lean, and may contain as much as 30% fat.

In fact the term 'meat' includes a very large range of products based on meat – sausages, hamburgers, ground meat products of various types, which may contain other foods, smoked meats like bacon, ham and pastrami, pickled meats, as well as poultry and game. They come from a variety of sources such as beef, veal, mutton, lamb, pork, horse, and more rarely buffalo, goat and many other animals. The nutrient content of the flesh of the various animals (except pig) is similar but the organs differ considerably [3].

In western countries meat products provide as much as one third of the average intake of protein and the same proportion of many of the B vitamins and of the iron, but since there are as many as forty types of products involved nutrient losses in any one process may be of little significance in the diet as a whole.

In poor diets based largely on cereals and root crops, meat plays a special rôle because, even if eaten in relatively small amounts, it makes a proportionately large contribution to the intake of B vitamins (meat is the only important source of vitamin B_{12}), the protein often complements the amino acid pattern of the staple food and, in particular, the iron of meat is well absorbed compared with any other food. This importance of the iron in meat holds even in well-fed western communities where anaemia is still a major nutritional disorder largely due to the poor absorption of the dietary iron from non-meat sources.

Hence, as discussed in the first chapter, the losses of nutrients in the various processes must be considered within the whole diet of the consumer.

Losses are of two kinds (*a*) loss of juices containing protein and B vitamins in solution, which are however, usually consumed; and (*b*) reduced availability of amino acids and partial destruction of thiamin. Clearly, the extent of the losses will vary with temperature, time and type of cooking, which in turn will depend, among other factors, on the size of the portion and its content of connective tissue.

There is a considerable difference between the temperature of the oven and the outer parts of a piece of meat on the one hand, and that of the inner parts on the other, depending on the conditions of heating and the composition and size of the portion. In stewing and canning the nutrients would be more thoroughly extracted but the extract would be eaten.

These many variables can account for differing results reported in the literature. Cover *et al.* (1949) [19] state that an internal temperature of 80°C will produce 'well done' beef, and 84°C for pork; this can be achieved with an oven temperature of 150°C. At high oven temperatures of 250°C the internal temperature can rise to 98°C – then the meat falls apart.

The important factor is that at the lower temperature there is a considerable amount of water-soluble nutrients in the meat juices which are edible, but at the higher temperature the juices become charred and inedible. In that case small amounts of protein and relatively large amounts of the B vitamins are destroyed.

Toepfer *et al.* (1955) [96a] cooked a variety of cuts of beef by oven roasting, pot roasting and griddle broiling from the frozen state. This involves losses in drips during thawing (thaw juices), consisting of protein and fat, the amount depends on the type of meat, ratio of area of cut surface to volume, and proportions of bone and fat.

Since the results came from one laboratory the comparison between different methods of cooking can be accepted as valid, even if they differ from those of other laboratories.

Broiling on a griddle without added fat lost 3% protein and 4% fat; braising Swiss steaks lost 16% protein and 40% fat. Cooking without water (oven roasts, griddle-broiled steaks, meat loaves, hamburgers) lost only 5% protein. Stewing lost 3% protein and no fat. Roasting lost 4% protein – 2.6% in thaw juice and 1.8% in pan drippings. Pot roasting, due to the addition of water, lost 10% protein, as well as 30% fat.

Pearson *et al.* (1950) [75] reported 10-15% loss of thiamin, riboflavin, niacin and folic acid in thaw juice, with 30% loss of pyridoxine.

Proteins

Apart from losses into juices proteins suffer little or no damage when meat is heated or processed under conditions that are similar to cooking procedures. Even at the higher temperatures reached during roasting it is only the outer parts that suffer damage and this is a small proportion of the total mass of meat. Such damage as does occur will include destruction in the dark crisped parts, and reduced availability of some of the amino acids through Maillard-type reactions. Since roasting is carried out in order to produce the desired flavour such loss of nutrients must presumably be regarded as a price worth paying.

Some articles and textbooks refer to the reduction of biological value consequent upon denaturation of proteins of meat during cooking. This is quite incorrect; denaturation does not affect protein quality (in any case, proteins are denatured in the stomach before digestion).

Beuk *et al.* (1948) [6] found that even after 24 h autoclaving at 112°C the only amino acid destroyed was cystine, but that PER was reduced from 3.2 to 2.6 after 2 h [7].

Mayfield and Hedrick (1949) [58] roasted meat in open pans at 163°C with an internal temperature of 80°C; they browned meat in the oven for 30 min then sterilised in the can, and they cured the meat with salt and found no change in nutritive value of the protein in any of the processes (although there was some discrepancy between pairs of assays).

In a range of meat products – bacon, pork, beef, chicken and shrimp – Thomas and Calloway (1961) found no losses of any of the essential amino acids when subjected to a variety of processing treatments including freeze-drying, cooking, canning and irradiation [547].

While most of the evidence quoted above indicates that meat suffers little or no damage when processed alone, there is evidence that heating in the presence of other foodstuffs does cause damage to the meat protein. Hellendoorn *et al.* (1971) [560] canned six types of meat dishes and examined their protein quality and vitamin contents after sterilisation, and also after 3 and 5 years subsequent storage.

| Sample | Percentage loss of protein quality | | |
| | Canning | Storage | |
		3 yr	5 yr
Goulash and potatoes	0	17	20
Spinach, pork and potatoes	12	16	20
Carrots, onions, beef and potatoes	18	25	31
Peas, minced meat and potatoes	0	15	24
Dun peas with bacon	30	33	40
White beans, bacon, potatoes and tomato sauce	+30	14	45

Two samples of the six showed no fall in NPU on canning, three showed losses of 12%, 18% and 30% respectively, and the sample containing white beans *increased* by 30%. This is presumably due to destruction of the toxins. All samples showed slow loss on storage.

Bender and Husaini (1976) [4] clearly showed that the damage was due to the presence of the other foodstuffs. Meat autoclaved alone was unchanged in protein quality but there was a fall due to the reduced availability of the sulphur amino acids when it was autoclaved in the presence of glucose and wheat flour (intended to simulate the commercial products canned with 'gravy').

Skurry and Osborne (1976) found a fall in the PER of a meat sausage on cooking but not in products in which the meat was party replaced with soya or milk solids. 'All-meat' sausages containing 7% cereal as a binder had PER 2.5 when raw, falling to 2.0 on cooking. When 60% of the meat was replaced by soya or milk solids the PER's were 1.4 and 1.7 respectively with no change on cooking [469].

Corned beef refers to different products in the United States (whole meat pickled in large pieces) and in Great Britain (a canned product made of partially extracted chopped beef, picked in the can). Mayfield and Hedrick (1949) [58] found no loss of protein quality in American corned beef (although there was some inconsistency in the assays), while Bender (1962) found that the NPU was 0.55 in the British product compared with 0.75 for fresh beef [751].

Pellett and Miller (1963) [76] found that traditional methods of preserving meat by salting and drying in the open air had little or no effect on protein quality. Biltong is made in Africa and the Middle East from long strips of muscle from cattle, sheep, goats and camels. The samples examined had suffered no loss with NPU 0.76 (sheep and goats) and 0.82 (cattle) compared with a laboratory dried sample of fresh meat at 0.80.

Charqui, produced usually from beef in South America, is salted and pressed before being dried and had NPU 0.67. Sucuk, traditional in the Middle East, is made by mincing, flavouring and drying in the air and the sample examined had NPU 0.72.

Vitamins

Thiamin is by far the most labile of the vitamins in meat, destruction depending on time and temperature, with smaller losses when high temperatures are involved for a shorter time. In pork, much richer than any other meat in thiamin, the vitamin appears to be more stable. As Table 8.1 shows losses of thiamin on braising beef are 40–50%, while from pork the loss is only 20–30%. Similarly, Cover et al. (1949) [19] found 30% loss from beef and 20% from pork roasted at the low temperature of 150°C (internal temperature 80°C). A small amount was in the drippings from beef, more in the pork drippings. Roasting at the higher temperature of 205°C (internal temperature 98°C) not only caused a greater destruction of thiamin in the meat but the drippings were charred and inedible with a total loss of 50% of thiamin from both types of meat.

In contrast the same authors found that pantothenate, niacin and riboflavin were relatively stable with no destruction (less than 10%) at 150°C – there was 20% of each vitamin in the drippings. At the higher temperature there was slightly greater extraction from the meat but since the drippings were charred there was overall 40% loss of pantothenate and 30% loss of niacin and riboflavin.

TABLE 8.1. Losses of thiamin in cooked meat (data from figures assembled by Farrer, 1955 [698])

		% loss
Beef:	roast	40–60
	broiled	50
	stewed	50 (up to 70)
	fried (variable conditions)	0–45
	braised	40–45
	canned (85 min at 121°C)	80
Pork:	braised	20–30
	roast	30–40
Ham:	baked	50
	fried	50
	broiled	20
	canned	50–60
Chop:	braised	15
Bacon:	fried	80
Mutton:	broiled chop	30–40
	roast leg	40–50
	stewed lamb	50
Poultry:	roast chicken, turkey	30–45
Fish:	fried	40

There is small loss during storage at low temperatures. Pork stored at −18°C lost 10–20% of the thiamin after 8 weeks, with no further loss after 48 weeks; riboflavin, 10–20% loss; pantothenate 0–10% loss; niacin, no loss.

There appear to be insignificant losses of thiamin when sliced meat is kept hot or reheated and kept hot [29].

Curing process

Curing and smoking of pork hams caused a loss of 20% of thiamin mostly during the smoking not the curing process; there was no loss of riboflavin or niacin [90, 80, 23].

On the other hand Hoagland *et al.* (1947) [39] reported that thiamin losses depended on the method of curing; artery-curing, dry-curing and brine-curing caused losses of 10%, 14% and 26% respectively. Protein quality was unchanged. Losses during subsequent storing also depended on the curing process.

There is a loss of B vitamins in bacon processing, 15% of thiamin in dry-cured bacon and 25% in wet-curing [41]. Differences were greater for riboflavin – 10% loss by wet-curing and 40% in dry-curing. No niacin was lost in dry-curing and 20% in wet-curing. Very little information appears to be available on the effects of curing and smoking meat products.

Canning

Meats canned in solid form without brine are subjected to greater heat during sterilisation than the liquid pack where the heat is transferred more rapidly. Thiamin is the only vitamin to suffer significant damage, various authors reporting losses between 15 and 30% [33].

Dehydration results in greater losses of B vitamins – 25% thiamin, 30% pantothenic acid, 8% niacin; no loss of riboflavin or biotin [81, 103].

Poultry

The only loss from pre-cooked frozen poultry is of thiamin – 40% loss on steaming 40 min, and a similar loss, (20–40%) on broiling [40, 66, 63]. There was little or no loss of riboflavin (variously reported as nil to 10–20% loss on broiling, frying, roasting or stewing).

Canning of chicken meat caused 70% loss of thiamin but no loss of riboflavin or niacin [63].

Roasting of turkeys, because of the longer time involved in larger pieces of tissue, results in greater loss. Two to 3 h roasting in an oven at 160°C resulted in 40% loss of thiamin from 'light meat', 70% from 'dark meat', 20–30% loss of riboflavin, 20–30% loss of niacin (17).

Polyunsaturated fats

Poultry fat is less saturated than that of beef and lamb, and ready-to-eat cooked chicken presents problems of rancidity on storage and subsequent reheating. The stability of both the cooking oil and the chicken lipids was examined in detail by Lee and Dawson (1973) [871].

Oils were examined after heating alone, with water-saturated cotton balls as a model and with chicken. Corn oil contained 59% linoleic acid, falling to 55% after 24 h heating at 200°C and after 48 h – the same values were found both in the oil heated alone or with cotton balls or chicken.

Chicken was cooked at 205°C for 9.5 min at 15 lb pressure and kept at 70°C for 15 min; fresh oil and oil previously heated for 24 and 48 h were examined.

The fat from raw chicken contained 24% linoleic acid, increasing to 34% on cooking due to pick-up from the oil with a slow fall during subsequent storage. The linoleic acid content of chicken stored raw fell from the initial value of 24% of the total fat, to 20% after 3 months and 16% after 6 months. Phospholipids, and neutral fats, and skin and meat separately, were also examined.

Oil previously heated for 42 h differed very little from fresh oil. The arachidonic acid content of the chicken fell on cooking in contrast to the linoleic acid, which rose, and after 6 months storage the total loss was 50%.

Offals

In contrast with meat (unless consumed immediately after slaughter) offals provide a source of vitamin C. Kizlaitis *et al.* (1964) [47] examined the effects of cooking at 76–93°C for 25 min on a variety of offals (heart, liver, brain, spleen, pancreas, tongue, kidney, thymus) and found losses of 10–50% – this included 25% passing into the drippings.

The only tissue that provided reasonable amounts of vitamin A was liver, and braising at an internal temperature of 170°C, caused losses of 0–10%; there were no drippings from the liver.

Storage

There is a difference in stability of vitamins in meats of different types and losses can occur even during the frozen stage. Pork chops stored for 6 months at −26°C lost 40% of the thiamin and 30% of the riboflavin but none of the niacin. In lamb stored under the same conditions the loss was only 20% of the thiamin; there was no loss at 3 months, while pork lost thiamin progressively [53, 54]. Cooking losses were additional to these storage losses.

Hams stored at 20°C for 32 weeks lost amounts of thiamin varying with the curing process; artery-cured ham lost 20%, dry-cured and brine-cured 30% [39].

Canned meat can lose thiamin during storage but the other B vitamins (riboflavin, niacin and pantothenate) are stable. Even at 37°C Rice and Robinson (1944) found no loss of riboflavin, niacin and pantothenate but canned pork lost half the thiamin after 43 weeks at 27°C. Thomas and Calloway (1961) [547] found small losses of riboflavin (zero to 10%) and niacin 5–15%) in canned meats stored 6 months at 38°C, but 40% loss of thiamin in 6 months at 38°C or 12 months at room temperature.

However, these small losses might have no statistical significance since the coefficient of variation reported by these authors was 50% for thiamin, 25% for riboflavin and 7% for niacin. Hence small or even moderate losses might remain undetected, or, alternatively, small apparent losses might be due to experimental error.

'Partially defatted meat'

Among processed meat products is one from which part of the fat has been removed, termed partially defatted chopped beef, and the residue is termed partially defatted beef fatty tissue. Both of these can be used in manufactured products (in the U.S.) such as frankfurters.

The beef is rendered at temperatures below 49°C; the partially defatted beef (PDB) is defined as containing at least 12% lean meat while the partially defatted tissue (FT) contains less than 12% lean meat. This compares with fatty tissue itself which consists of 85–93% fat, 6–13% water and only 2–3% protein [36].

Protein efficiency ratio of PDB was between 1.1 and 2.6 compared with 2.85 for beef, the value depends on the amount of connective tissue present since this is extremely low in sulphur amino content. For example three samples of PDB had (a) PER 2.85, with collagen 12.8%; (b) 2.58, with collagen 20.7% and (c) 1.16, with collagen 40%. Samples of FT in which the small amount of protein is largely collagen, had PER 1.7, with collagen 45% and 1.13, with collagen 50%.

FISH

Fish is mainly of value as a source of protein and iodine, and fatty fish is of considerable importance as one of the few dietary sources of vitamin D. It is a minor and unimportant source of a range of the B vitamins.

Canning softens the bones and renders them edible so they become, as are small fish that are eaten whole, a useful source of calcium. This may be included as one of the beneficial effects of processing.

Fatty fish may also be important as a source of polyunsaturated fatty acids ($C_{20:5}$ and $C_{22:6}$).

Most of the investigations of the effects of processing have been devoted to protein damage in fish meal used for animal feed and, in more recent years, to fish protein concentrate intended for human food. Little information is available of the effects on the vitamin D, the iodine and the polyunsaturated fatty acids in the wide variety of processes in common use such as smoking, drying, salting, and canning.

Since fish is so perishable a product preservation is a matter of considerable importance especially in developing countries, where it can make a major contribution to the diet. Traditional methods, such as smoking and drying, are often carried out under extremely variable conditions sometimes resulting in partly decomposed and partly charred material. Little is known of such effects on nutritional value but the few reports available indicate that smoking can protect the fats and that sometimes the damage to the protein on drying is less than in industrialised factories. Daun (1975) quotes reports of reactions between smoke products and sulphydryl and amino groups and available lysine [603].

Protein

Fish proteins are limited by the sulphur amino acids and contain a relative surplus of lysine so that damage to the latter may have no effect on NPU. Hake fillets dried at 105°C, for example, showed no change in NPU despite a fall in available lysine from 8.6 to 6.9% [149], nor was any change found on canning sardines [148].

Tooley and Lawrie (1974) [146] reported a fall of 20–30% in available lysine when white fish (cod, haddock, coley, plaice and skate) were fried in a variety of fresh vegetable oils. This increased to 40% when overheated ('thermally abused') oils were used. Damage was apparently due to the formation of linkages between the amino groups of the protein and oxidation products of the fat since it was much less when the fish was coated with batter before frying, so providing a barrier.

Pieniazek et al. (1975) [817] measured the available sulphur amino acids in heated mackerel. At 115°C available cystine fell to 35% and at 126°C to 25% of the initial value, with no change in total cystine. Methionine was more stable – there was no change at 115°C and a reduction of 20% of the available methionine at 126°C. Steaming had no effect on the availability of either of these amino acids (Table 4.1).

De Groot (1963) examined a fish pattie mixture of cooked haddock with cornmeal, fat and flavourings fried for 2.5 min at 200°C; BV fell from 0.87 to 0.83; digestibility was unaffected [533].

Most of the investigations reported in the literature have involved fish meal intended for animal feed and the relatively severe and often uncontrolled processing causes damage to the sulphur amino acids with considerable falls in NPU.

Among less common types of treatment of fish is the preparation of Bombay duck (*Harpoden nehereus*) reported by Sen *et al.* (1969) [139]. The material was sun-dried, shredded and extracted with ethanol, or cooked, pressed and dried then extracted with ethanol. The authors found no loss of lysine or sulphur amino acids compared with fresh fish but reported a loss of tryptophan by microbiological assay; BV was not measured.

Other nutrients

Most white fish are relatively poor sources of vitamins and so losses are of lesser importance. There is no loss on cooking – but drying can result in 50% loss of thiamin and 65% loss of riboflavin [109]. Thiamin is also unstable to irradiation, up to 50% being lost when treated with 0.6 Mrad, with an additional loss of 10% on cooking. Riboflavin is more stable, the combined losses on irradiation and cooking being 15%; niacin was not affected [120].

TABLE 8.2. Loss of thiamin from fish subjected to various heat treatments (frozen fish and batter and breading mix initially 0.25 mg thiamin/100 g) (Ang *et al.*, 1975 [574])

	% loss
Heat in convection oven	
held 0.5 h	0
1.5 h	10
3.0 h	20
* Heat infrared oven	
held 0.5 h	5
Steamer	
held 0.5 h	10
Microwave	
held 0.5 h	5

* To simulate convenience food systems handling.

Table 8.2 shows the small losses of thiamin from fish with batter cooked in a variety of ways [574].

Canning and subsequent storage cause negligible damage but there can be considerable extraction into the canning brine or sauce of fat, fat-soluble vitamins and bone minerals. These, of course, are lost if the liquor is discarded.

The vitamin of greatest importance in fish is vitamin D in fatty species and this appears to be stable to canning, freezing and smoke-curing although evidence is scarce.

Iodine was shown to be very largely destroyed by freezing and 30–40% destroyed by salting and smoking (see p. 82).

The polyunsaturated fatty acids in hake and sea bream were not affected by boiling (25–30 min) or roasting (220–240°C for 40–50 min). Some other varieties of fish did suffer a loss, for example dusky sea bream lost 20% both on boiling and on roasting. The $C_{22:6}$ chain fatty acids appeared to increase on boiling [137].

Solvents

Solvent treatment of fish meal in the preparation of fish protein concentrates and isolates can reduce nutritional value or give rise to toxic products arising from residues of the solvent. Prolonged solvent treatment, 24 h at 83°C, produced fish protein concentrate that would not support growth and contained as much as 30 000 ppm dichloroethane. At the slightly lower temperature of 65°C for the same length of time the residual solvent was much less (2000 ppm) and growth rate was near maximal, little less than material treated at 40°C with residual solvent at 17 ppm [779].

MILK

Milk is an extremely valuable source of many nutrients, particularly of protein of high biological value, calcium and riboflavin, as well as vitamin A, a range of B vitamins and, in the raw state, of vitamin C. However, it is a highly perishable product and can be a source of infection so that some degree of processing is almost always essential. Some destruction of nutrients is inevitable, although less with modern treatment than with older methods. This serves as an example of a price worth paying for safety, quite apart from the obvious point that the unprocessed product might be completely wasted.

Milk undergoes a great variety of processes, some of which are discussed below, and the loss of nutrients depends largely on exposure to light, and the time and intensity of heat treatment, together with the presence of oxygen. The subject has been reviewed by Kon (1961) and Gregory (1975) [195, 175].

Effect of light

As much as 50% of the riboflavin in milk can be destroyed in 2 h if exposed to bright sunshine in a bottle; even on a dull day this can be 20%. The riboflavin is converted into lumichrome and lumiflavine, which then destroy the vitamin C present. The destruction of a small part of the riboflavin – as little as 5% – can catalyse large-scale destruction of the vitamin C – as much as 90%. An unpleasant flavour – 'sunlight-flavour' – can also develop, possibly due to the formation of methional by reaction between methionine and riboflavin, and also to oxidation of fat [151, 181, 200, 209].

Grudskaja (1965) [179a] showed that the vitamin C was far more stable when the milk was protected by coloured glass – in 2 h it was completely destroyed in clear glass bottles, and the loss was reduced to 10% in dark green bottles and to 4% in brown bottles. Clearly, pigmented glass would be advantageous but appears to have negative sales appeal.

This effect of sunlight has been known for many years but was re-examined when it became common practice to offer milk for sale in cartons in supermarkets where it was exposed to fluorescent light. This causes destruction of vitamin C and development of a 'light flavour' even in fibreboard cartons. The flavour could be detected after only 20 min in clear glass bottles, after 5 h in amber glass and after 1–15 h in various types of fibreboard cartons [165].

The destruction of riboflavin and vitamin C was directly related to the radiant power emitted between wavelengths of 400 and 550 nm but the same relation did not hold for the development of the flavour.

Hedrick and Glass (1975) [181] examined the effects of fluorescent light on milk in plastic or paperboard containers exposed for 5, 10 and 24 h. Vitamin C was very unstable in plastic containers, 30%, 45% and 95% being destroyed at the three respective times of exposure. It was more stable in paperboard, the corresponding figures being 7, 15 and 45%. Even when kept in the dark there was a loss of 50% in 10 days in plastic containers and 40% in paperboard.

Riboflavin, however, was little affected under these conditions, losses being 0 to 7% in plastic and 0 to 4% in paperboard after 24 h. This confirms the earlier finding that small changes in riboflavin catalyse large losses of vitamin C. Singh *et al.* (1975) [209] also found very little loss of riboflavin in normal polythene containers and no loss when gold-pigmented polythene or paperboard cartons were used.

When riboflavin has been subjected to light in the presence of oxygen it affects the milk proteins by increasing the coagulation time [175].

Vitamin B$_6$

In raw milk this is present as pyridoxal, which is converted into the amine during sterilisation. On storage the pyridoxamine complexes with sulphur compounds leading to the formation of bis-4-pyridoxyl disulphide which has much lower biological activity (in rats).

When milk is autoclaved at high temperatures a large part of the vitamin B_6 can be destroyed. It was the introduction of such a process that gave rise to clinical signs of B_6 deficiencies in babies, and first established this vitamin as a dietary essential for human beings. The loss is probably due to reaction with -SH groups of the protein since pyridoxine is stable when heated alone [714].

Temperature differences may explain the contradictory reports of the stability of vitamin B_6 during sterilisation and drying. Table 8.3, which is a summary of the experience of the National Institute for Research in Dairying, Shinfield, England, shows graded losses from 50% with older methods of in-bottle sterilisation, to 20% with newer in-bottle methods and finally to less than 10% loss by UHT sterilisation. When others have reported losses of 40–60% on sterilisation (Hassinen *et al.*, 1954) these have presumably been incurred under severe conditions. Similarly Burton *et al.* (1967), also of the National Institute for Research in Dairying, reported a loss of 30% of vitamin B_6 by in-bottle sterilisation at 110°C for 20 min.

Variations in conditions may also explain why Ford *et al.* (1974) [171] reported B_6 to be stable to drying while Srncova and Davidek (1972) [714] found 50–85% loss in a number of samples of dried milk.

Pasteurisation

This is the commonest treatment to which milk is subjected and is intended to destroy all pathogens and many other organisms except thermoduric and thermophilic ones. The heat process must be followed by rapid cooling to retard the growth of the remaining organisms. A number of enzymes are also destroyed – amylase, catalase, lipase, peroxidase, phosphatase, xanthine oxidase – which, if allowed to persist, would cause undesirable flavours to develop.

The time needed for the destruction of undesirable organisms is inversely proportional to the temperature, and this has brought about two main methods of pasteurisation, a longer time at a low temperature (the old holder method; 62°C for 30 min) or a high temperature for a short time (HTST; 72°C for 15 s). Since biological systems are more sensitive to temperature than are chemical systems such as those involved in damage to nutrients, HTST is preferred both organoleptically and nutritionally.

The most sensitive nutrients are vitamins C and B_1; vitamins A and D are not affected, see Table 8.3.

TABLE 8.3. Typical values for the proportion of heat-labile vitamins in raw milk lost during heat treatment (Porter and Thompson, 1976 [202a])

Milk	Thiamin	Vitamin B$_6$	Vitamin B$_{12}$	Folic acid	Vitamin C
Pasteurised	<0.10	<0.10	<0.10	<0.10	<0.25
In-bottle sterilised:					
old method	0.35	0.50	0.90	0.50	0.90
new method	0.20	0.20	0.20	0.30	0.60
UHT sterilised	<0.10	<0.10	<0.10	<0.10	<0.25
Evaporated	0.20	0.40	0.80	0.25	0.60
Sweetened-condensed	0.10	<0.10	0.30	0.25	0.25

Apart from specific effects on vitamins there are slight changes in the minerals – a small decrease in soluble calcium and soluble phosphate.

Sterilisation

Since this requires a higher temperature than pasteurisation there is considerable destruction of vitamins C, B$_{12}$, B$_6$, folate and thiamin, but losses can be reduced by increasing the temperature and decreasing the time (Ultra-high temperature – UHT) as shown in Table 8.3. Nearly all of the vitamin C present in the dehydro form, about one-quarter of the total, is lost, but there are only small losses of folate, vitamin B$_6$ and B$_{12}$. Since these losses are largely due to dissolved oxygen they can be reduced to insignificant amounts by de-aeration before heating. Thiamin, vitamin A and carotene are stable, see Table 8.4 [157]. De-aeration also allows long storage with little loss of vitamins (Table 8.5).

The overall effect of UHT treatment is that milk can be preserved for many months with about the same loss of nutrients as incurred in pasteurisation.

TABLE 8.4. Loss of vitamins (per cent loss of initial value) in UHT sterilised milk (oxygen content 9 ppm) (Burton *et al.*, 1970 [157])

	Indirect heat (141°C)	Direct heat (144°C)
Vitamin C	8	8
Dehydroascorbic acid	80	85
Vitamin B$_1$	0	0
Folate	4–19	0–13
Vitamin B$_6$	10	6
Vitamin B$_{12}$	4	13
Vitamin A	0	0
Carotene	0	0

TABLE 8.5. Relationship between loss of vitamins during storage and oxygen content of UHT milk (Burton *et al.*, 1970 [157])

	Initial oxygen level (ppm)	Period of storage (days)	Loss during storage (%)
Ascorbic acid	0.1	60	20
	1–2	14	100
	8	7	100
Folic acid	0.1	60	0
	1–2	60	5
	8	14	100
Vitamin B$_{12}$	0.1 ⎫ 1–2 ⎬ 8 ⎭	60	25–60

Evaporation

Evaporated milk is defined according to the U.S. Standards of Identity as containing not less than 7.9% milk fat and not less than 25.9% total solids; stabiliser and vitamin D may be added.

During the concentration process there is a darkening of the colour, partly due to concentration of solids and of carotene but also to Maillard reaction. Since milk proteins are limited by the sulphur amino acids the damage, unless severe, is not revealed by NPU assay. Mauron *et al.* (1955) [197] showed 8% destruction of lysine together with a further 12% fall in available lysine (Table 8.6). Vitamin losses in evaporation are considerable (Table 8.3).

'Condensed milk' usually contains 28% milk solids with 8.5% fat; skimmed condensed milk is sweetened and preserved by the addition of sucrose. This allows preservation with less heat and consequently less damage to the nutrients (Table 8.3).

Lactose can crystallise out of condensed milk during prolonged storage but there is no other change.

Vitamins A, D and niacin are not affected. Damage to riboflavin appears to be variable according to different authors but this may be due to light rather than heat.

Drying

Both skim and full cream milk are dried to about 5% moisture; folic acid, thiamin and vitamin B$_6$ appear to be quite stable but there can be a loss of 40% of the riboflavin [171].

Available lysine is not affected by spray drying but there is a loss of both total and available lysine in roller drying and this can be considerable if processing conditions are not adequately controlled (Table 8.6).

For example Erbersdobler and Zucker (1966) [168] reported losses in commercial roller-dried samples of 40% available lysine and as much as 50% in material dried on rollers manufactured before 1960. The loss was confirmed by bioassay which indicates that the protein had been damaged sufficiently to reduce the available lysine below the levels of methionine and cystine which are normally the limiting amino acids.

TABLE 8.6. Total and available lysine content (g/16 g nitrogen) of milk and milk products (Mauron *et al.*, 1955 [197])

Type of milk	Lysine Content	
	Total	Available
Fresh	8.3	8.0
Spray-dried powder	8.0	7.9
Evaporated	7.6	6.7
Roller-dried powders:		
commercial	7.1	6.0
slightly scorched	6.2	4.0

If protected from moisture dried milk is stable to prolonged storage, both organoleptically and nutritionally. Eggum *et al.* (1970) [166] stored milk powder in paper bags in a barn for a year at temperatures varying between $-11°C$ and $+48°C$ and at RH between 24 and 100%. There was a small fall in NPU (from 0.74 to 0.71) and in digestibility (from 92% to 90%); control samples kept at $-20°C$ remained unchanged at NPU 74. There was a fall in lysine of 7% and in methionine plus cystine from 3.36 to 2.94 g/16 g N.

The instantisation process for dried skim milk has no effect on the B vitamins and only a small effect on vitamin C [195].

Moore and Williams (1965) [198] found that the commercial drying process had no effect on the linoleic and arachidonic acid content of milk but pointed out that these fatty acids may have been isomerised, a change which would not be revealed by their methods, and that this may explain why their results differed from those of Pol and Groot (1960) who found a 30–40% loss [201].

Other methods of preservation

Milk can be preserved by the addition of hydrogen peroxide (Buddeization) followed by its removal with catalase, and apart from almost complete destruction of the vitamin C the process has very little effect on nutritive value [195, 178]. No other vitamins were damaged and there was a reduction of 6% in protein quality.

Ultraviolet light has the double effect of both increasing the vitamin D content and reducing the bacterial count by up to 70–80%. There is no nutritional loss [195].

One Mrad of ionising radiation can destroy up to two-thirds of both retinol and carotene, half the vitamin E, 90% of the C and the thiamin, 75% of the riboflavin, 80% of the vitamin B_6 and 'some' of the niacin [195].

In many countries the only method available of preserving milk is by curdling and there is a great variety of traditional soured milks. The only loss appears to be thiamin – Pasricha (1969) [199] reported an average loss of 60% (ranging between 40% and 100%) in buffalo milk treated with a variety of bacterial cultures used domestically in India. The process involved boiling, cooling and incubating with the inoculum for 15 h. Losses of riboflavin were so small and variable as to be considered negligible. There is considerable variability between different reports, no doubt reflecting differences in procedure, and some of these indicate loss of part of the retinol and B vitamins.

CEREALS

Cereals provide about three-quarters of both the energy and the protein of human diets; even in western countries where a wide variety of foods is available this proportion is still about one quarter.

When one cereal provides the main part of the diet its nutritional quality plays a dominant role in the health of the community. It does not matter to the vast majority of western populations whether their rice is white, brown or enriched but a high death rate from beri-beri has long been associated with diets in which polished rice forms the greater part, just as pellagra is common where maize is the staple food.

In their unrefined state wheat at 10% protein, rice at 8%, and even the poorer of the millets at 6–14% protein supply adequate protein and B vitamins, at least for adults. It is when the grain has been milled and a large proportion of the vitamins and a smaller proportion of the protein are discarded that the food becomes inadequate.

Storage

One of the virtues of cereals is that they can be stored for many years so long as the moisture content is not too high. For example, there was no loss of thiamin from rice after two year's storage when the moisture was below 10% [220, 241, 264] nor from maize. After 2.5 years white rice lost 30% thiamin, 5% riboflavin and niacin; brown rice lost a little less thiamin [262].

Caileau *et al.* (1945) [228] examined brown rice, white rice, bran and polishings and reported a loss of 30% of the thiamin after 6 months storage

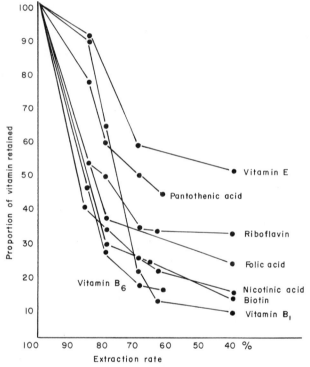

FIG. 8.1. The relationship between extraction rate and proportion of the total vitamins of the grain retained in flour. (Moran, 1959 [274])

at 20°C. After 24 months the losses were 50–70%. Canned and parboiled brown rice and parboiled undermilled rice lost little or nothing after 6 months storage.

In one series of observations wheat stored at the high moisture content of 17% lost 30% of its thiamin in 5 months; at the normal moisture content of 12% the loss was 12%; at very low moisture content, 6%, there was no loss after one year's storage [241].

Thiamin-enriched flour lost 10% of the vitamins after 6 months storage under 'normal' conditions and 20% under 'unfavourable' conditions [703]. The riboflavin and niacin appear to be quite stable.

Vitamin A is present in yellow maize largely as cryptoxanthin and this is unstable particularly in milled grain even in cool storage. When stored whole in steel bins half of the vitamin A potency was lost after 4 years (Jones *et al.*, 1943) [936] but after milling losses were as much as one-third in one week at 35°C (Fraps and Kemmerer, 1937) [937]. Zeleny (in Harris and van Loesecke [895]) reported a study of maize crops between 1937 and 1941 with losses as high as 70% after one year's storage 'under Government seal' (i.e. presumably good storage conditions).

TABLE 8.7. Loss of nutrients in milling of wheat (content per 100 g) (McCance and Widdowson, 1960 [909], Moran, 1959 [274])

Percentage extraction	100	85	80	70	45
Protein (g)	13.6	13.6	13.2	12.8	11.8
Fat (g)	2.5	1.7	1.4	1.2	0.9
Fibre (g)	2.2	0.3	0.1		
Thiamin (mg)	0.4	0.35	0.25	0.08	0.03
Niacin (mg)	5.0	2.0	1.6	1.1	0.7
Riboflavin (mg)	0.16	0.08	0.08	0.05	0.02
Pantothenate (mg)	1.5	1.1	0.9	0.7	
Pyridoxine (mg)	0.4	0.18	0.11	0.06	
Biotin (μg)	5.0		1.4	1.1	0.7
Folate (μg)	35	18	13		8

The moisture content of the cereal will depend on conditions at the time of harvesting. Chow and Draper (1969) found that when maize was dried down from 25% to 15% moisture content there was no effect on the fatty acids or the tocopherol [235].

Milling

The major processing losses in cereals are due to milling since the bran and germ are discarded.

Figure 8.1 and Table 8.7 show the effects of milling of wheat on thiamin, niacin, riboflavin, folic acid, pantothenate, vitamin B_6 and vitamin E. Obviously, the more highly milled the grain, i.e. the larger the amount discarded, (the lower the extraction rate), the greater is the loss of nutrients. It is necessary to strike a balance between palatibility, convenience and nutritional value and this has become, in many countries, a matter of national policy together with restoration of part of the milling losses.

Thiamin occurs mostly in the scutellum portion of the germ and in the aleurone layer. Oats differ from most other cereals in having a higher proportion of thiamin in the bran and aleurone layer than in the endosperm.

Riboflavin is more evenly spread throughout the grain although there is more in the germ and aleurone layer; niacin mostly occurs in the aleurone layer with little in the germ; vitamin E is found mostly in the germ.

Since cereals are an important source of thiamin and niacin in most diets, processing losses can be a serious matter and in many countries some of the nutrients such as iron, thiamin and niacin are restored to white flour. At the same time bread is a useful vehicle for enrichment and calcium and riboflavin are sometimes added.

Apart from the loss of nutrients in the discarded bran and germ the lipids in rice are more susceptible to oxidation after milling [291]. There was no lipid oxidation in unmilled rice stored 3 years at ambient temperatures in the dark but rancidity developed after only a few months in milled and also parboiled rice. This was attributed to destruction of antioxidants and to mechanical damage during milling which exposed the fat to the air.

Rice

Rice serves as an outstanding example of the serious consequences of food processing, even though it is the traditional method that is the cause of the trouble rather than modern technology.

For thousands of years the rice grain has been extracted from the husk by pounding in a wooden or stone mortar. The outer husk is broken and separated from the grain by winnowing but some of the germ and the pericarp are removed at the same time, the amount depending on the treatment. Machine milling can produce a highly refined product with even greater loss of the bran. Husked rice may contain about 4 μg thiamin/g rice; once polished, 1.8, twice polished 1.0, and thrice polished (ready for sale – about 80% extraction rate) as little as 0.7 μg/g [218], see Table 8.8 [254]. There is simultaneously a loss of other B vitamins but in areas of the world where polished rice is the staple food it is the thiamin deficiency that is most severe and results in beri-beri – at one time a major cause of death in many countries.

A nutritionally better method of processing is parboiling before milling – the unhusked rice is soaked in water then steamed or boiled and dried before being husked. This has the double effect of causing part of the B vitamins to migrate into the inner part and also making it easier to remove the husk without as much loss of bran. The grain is partially gelatinised, less easily damaged in milling and keeps better during storage. The milled product contains up to 2 μg thiamin per g compared with only 0.7 in the untreated grain [218].

Parboiling is a traditional process in many countries but it suffers the disadvantages of changing the colour, taste and odour compared with polished white rice. So although it may be nutritionally desirable to recommend consumption of parboiled rice it is often not accepted. The factory equivalent process is 'converted rice' which includes vacuum treatment during soaking, steaming under pressure and continuous processing, (Malek, Garibaldi and Fernandez processes) resulting in better colour, taste and odour.

TABLE 8.8. Vitamin content of rice (mg/100 g) (Houston and Kohler, 1970 [254])

	B_1	B_2	Niacin	B_6	Pantothenate	Folate
Brown rice	0.34	0.05	4.7	1	1.5	0.02
Milled	0.07	0.03	1.6	0.45	0.75	0.02
Bran	2.26	0.25	30	2.5	2.8	0.15
Polishings	1.84	0.18	28	2.0	3.3	0.19
Germ	6.5	0.5	3.3	1.6	3.0	0.43

Earlier work [261] showed that the vitamin content of converted rice is much superior to that of polished rice and the same as that of parboiled rice. Thiamin is five times as high, niacin and B_6 three times, riboflavin, pantothenate and biotin are double, and folate is slightly greater.

Protein quality appears to be slightly improved although this may not be a significant change, especially since the assays were carried out under unconventional conditions, i.e. PER was measured on a 5% protein diet fed for 70 days and BV also on 5% protein diet [261]. Under these conditions PER improved both on parboiling and on 'converting' from 1.4 to 1.7; BV increased from 0.82 to 0.87 with a slight fall in digestibility making the NPU increase from 0.78 to 0.81. Even if the improvement is not significant the results do demonstrate that treatment did not damage the protein.

Recent work [280] showed a change in the structure of the rice granules, protein bodies and fat globules with parboiling, so that on milling there is a slightly greater loss of protein and fat since the bran contains 14–15% protein instead of 13% from uncooked rice, and 17–20% fat compared with 15–16%. However, as the figures in Table 8.9 show, despite some loss of thiamin during the parboiling process the final material contains much more thiamin. Calculated as thiamin per 1000 kcal of energy from the food, the parboiled rice is adequate in B vitamins. There is no loss of niacin or riboflavin during parboiling and greater retention afterwards. These authors explain some of the contradictions in the literature by the difficulty of milling constant fractions from different samples of parboiled rice.

There are also reports of losses of thiamin from rice by leaching into the washing and cooking water. However, as discussed under Thiamin (p. 34), Roy and Rao (1963) [285] showed that this was not due to leaching but to destruction through alkalinity of the water. They found no loss on cooking in distilled water compared with 36% loss on cooking in well water. Rice cooked in 10–15 volumes of well water (rice gruel) lost 80% compared with only 5% in distilled water.

TABLE 8.9. Thiamin in rice (μg/g). (Padua and Juliano, 1974 [280])

		Whole	Milled
Variety 1	brown rice	3.2	0.45
	parboiled (traditional method*)	2.5	1.9
Variety 2	brown rice	3.9	0.5
	commercially parboiled	2.8	2.1
Variety 3	brown rice	3.8	0.6
	treated 100°C	3.6	0.95
	treated 121°C	3.2	2.9
Variety 4	brown rice	3.7	0.6
	parboiled	3.6	1.8

* Hot water soak.

Heat damage

Cereals in general are not damaged when cooked in water, it is only when higher temperatures are reached that there is destruction of thiamin and loss of available lysine. High temperatures can be reached on the dry outside, for example, of a loaf of bread, while the moist inside is still below the boiling point of water. The temperature of the inside of foods such as biscuits will depend on the amount of moisture left. Mossman *et al.* (1973) [275] heated wheat flour at 327°C for periods of 10 to 40 s so controlling the moisture content and internal temperature of the product. At moisture levels of 20–30% the thiamin fell from 1.5 to 1.1 mg per lb; at 10% moisture it fell to 0.4 mg.

Protein quality was unchanged after 15 s heating while the moisture content was 20%, but PER fell from 1.27 to 0.88 after 40 s heating.

As discussed under Proteins (p. 65), one of the main factors is the presence of reducing substances causing loss of available lysine. Halevy and Guggenheim (1953) [791] found no change when wheat gluten was heated alone, but in the presence of glucose BV fell from 0.55 to 0.18. Addition of lysine restored the value to 0.63 (this is a higher value than initially since lysine was the limiting amino acid in the unheated material).

A similar example was provided by Block *et al.* (1946) [757a] who studied the effect of heat on a cake mix consisting of flour, egg, yeast and lactalbumin. The raw material had PER 3.5, which fell to 2.4 when baked for 15–20 min at 200°C, and to 0.8 when toasted for 40–60 min at 130°C. Again, addition of lysine restored the initial value.

Bread

Vitamins

Baking destroys 15–30% of the thiamin of bread with no loss of riboflavin or niacin; there is no further loss on storage [239, 306].

Reported losses of thiamin in making chappatis range from zero to 73%.

Farrer (1955) [698] emphasised the conflict of evidence in the literature regarding the losses of thiamin in different types of bread, depending on extraction rates, whether the thiamin was free, bound as cocarboxylase or protein bound, and the presence of mineral salts.

Obviously time and temperature influence the extent of the losses but in some baked goods pH is an important factor. Thiamin is relatively stable below pH 7, but a considerable amount is destroyed at alkaline pH. Briant and Klosterman (1950) [225] showed losses of 15% at pH 6.0 and 6.4, 25% at pH 6.9, 55% at pH 7.5, and 95% at pH 9.1.

In order to investigate chappatis Chaudri and Muller (1974) [234] studied 100 g dough discs of 15 cm diameter, dusted with 1.5 g flour, and baked 4 min, with regular turning. At a time-averaged temperature of 257°C, halving the thickness increased a thiamin loss of 20% to 60%.

Toasting bread is a variable process; in one series of observations toasting for periods of 30–70 s destroyed 10–30% of the thiamin [244]. Slices 9 mm and 12 mm thick lost 14% of the thiamin, increasing to 30% in 5 mm slices [239].

Cakes lost 23% of their thiamin increasing to 33% when self-raising baking powder was used [239].

Folic acid is partly destroyed during baking – Keagy *et al* (1973) [259] reported that one-third of the folate naturally present but only 10% of the added folate were destroyed (see p. 41).

Protein

Damage to protein occurs mainly through loss of available lysine, although loss of tryptophan has also been reported [249]. The interior of a loaf never reaches 100°C, however hot the oven, so it is the crust rather than the crumb that is damaged. However, the crust is only a small part of the whole, depending on the size and shape of the loaf, so that the total damage is small.

In one series of measurements there was a 10% reduction in protein quality, three-quarters of which was in the crumb [249, 284].

An investigation of the effects of baking was carried out by Gotthold and Kennedy (1964) [250] using PER, biological value by the Thomas–Mitchell nitrogen balance method, NPU by carcass analysis and digestibility. Wholemeal wheat flour was steamed for 20 min or baked at 218°C for 25 min. A 10-day PER assay showed a significant fall from a value of 1.3 on the raw ingredients, to 1.0 on steaming and 0.8 on baking. A 28-day PER assay showed no loss on steaming and a fall from 1.6 to 1.3 on baking. Biological value fell from 0.59 to 0.54 on baking which was statistically significant (steamed bread was not examined); digestibility fell from 95% to 92%, NPU, which combines both BV and digestibility, fell from a value of 0.51 in the ingredients to 0.48 on steaming and 0.43 on baking. Although the different assay methods do not agree one must conclude that there is a small loss in digestibility and BV on steaming and a slightly greater loss on baking.

Since wheat flour is limited in protein quality by its lysine content synthetic lysine is sometimes added. A biological study showed that added lysine was lost progressively during baking times up to 50 min; 30 min at 232°C caused a loss of 30% [258]. Lysine present as the free amino acid was no more sensitive to treatment than the protein-bound lysine.

Alternatively, skim milk powder may be used to supplement the lysine. The presence of extra reducing sugars from added milk powder or even the addition of sucrose at high enough concentration, as in biscuits, increased the rate of loss of lysine (determined chemically [236] – see under Biscuits (p. 147)).

There is a report [252] that the availability of several of the essential amino acids (methionine, tryptophan and leucine) is increased when flour is baked into bread but the finding that there was also an increase when the wheat was milled (isoleucine increasing by as much as 25%) suggests that further investigation is required.

During staling bread can lose a further 10–15% of the available lysine; toasting, varying, of course, with severity of treatment, can cause a loss of 5–10% [284].

These losses occur in the European-type loaves, cubic or spherical in shape, usually baked at 250°C for 45 min, with an internal temperature of about 95°C. Maleki and Djazayeri (1968) found no loss in an Arab-type of bread which was baked in a 1 cm layer for only 1 min at 400–500°C [269].

Methods of baking

Among the modern changes in methods of processing is the Chorleywood Bread Process, first introduced into the baking industry in 1961 and now widespread. This has also involved the use of specially developed wheat flours. However, there is little or no difference between this and conventionally made breads [263] – thiamin, available nicotinic acid, vitamin B_6, free folate, protein quality, fat and minerals were the same. There was slightly less protein in the Chorleywood bread – 132 g compared with 137 g protein per kg dry wt (probably due to the different flours used). Riboflavin, very low in flour in any case, was statistically higher in Chorleywood bread – 0.4 mg compared with 0.3 mg/kg dry wt.

The ascorbic acid used in this process – 75 ppm of flour – is completely destroyed during baking [298]. Using radioactive materials 30% was shown to be lost as CO_2, 25% left in the bread as L-threonic acid and smaller amounts of 2,3-diketogulonic acid together with a number of other breakdown products.

Another development in bread making is the Continuous Dough-mix which Toepfer *et al.* (1972) [300] examined. The vitamin content was the same as in bread made by conventional methods except for a slight fall in riboflavin.

Biscuits

Biscuits are baked to a lower moisture content and therefore a higher internal temperature than bread with consequently more severe damage. Proncuk *et al.* (1973) showed a fall of 72% in NPU between raw materials and biscuits baked at 180°C for 13 min [819].

Normally, biscuits are not an important part of the diet so that processing losses might be ignored but they do offer an attractive vehicle for nutrient enrichment, especially for children – protein, amino acids, vitamins and minerals can readily be incorporated without much change in texture and flavour, biscuits are stable to storage and they are convenient for a child to eat. However, the baking losses must be taken into account.

Supplementation with skim milk to produce a high protein biscuit in Uganda demonstrated part of the problem [237]. The available lysine fell from 4 g to 2 g per 16 g nitrogen due to linkage with the lactose of the skim milk; when the milk powder was replaced with casein there was no loss. Clark *et al.* (1959) [236] baked biscuits at 232°C and found no loss of available lysine after 10 min, 9% loss after 20 min, 18% loss after 25 min, and 27% after 30 min. The addition of sugar up to 14.5% had no effect on the lysine but when the sugar level was 29% there was a loss of available lysine in 20 min, i.e. three times the loss in the absence of sugar. With 58% sugar the loss was 65%. Added synthetic lysine was lost at the same rate.

High protein biscuits baked at 260–290°C showed losses in protein quality depending on the addition of malt or corn syrup, which supplied reducing sugars. Two biscuits showed a fall in PER from 2.2 to 1.4 and from 2.0 to 1.6, while another without sugars fell from 2.5 to 2.2 [282].

As frequently found, the commercial equivalent samples showed much greater damage; an over-baked biscuit, very dark brown in colour, had PER of only 1.0.

Breakfast cereals

Manufactured breakfast cereals are subjected to a variety of treatments and have been examined for protein damage [251, 265, 276, 294, 295, 305, 812].

The heating, rolling and flaking processes do not affect the protein, it is the more severe process of 'explosion' puffing that reduces the nutritive value. Rolled oats showed no change when boiled for 15 min and dried at

TABLE 8.10. Nutritive value of U.S. breakfast cereals (tested on rats) (from Sure, 1951 [295])

	Protein content (%)	Protein efficiency ratio
Quick Oats	17	1.6
Instant Ralston	13.8	1.5
Cerevim	18	1.5
Pablum	15	1.3
Cream of Wheat	11.2	1.2
Cheerios	14.9	1.1
Bran Flakes	9.5	0
Grape Nuts	9.2	−0.3
Kix	7.8	−0.9
Puffed Wheat	13.2	−2.5

130°C for 15 s or even when cooked for 1–2 min at 100 lb pressure, exploded and dried at 200°C for 1–2 min. When, however, oats were puffed by heating for 5 min at 122°C, then heated at 200 lb pressure at 189°C for 2 min there was a fall in PER from the original value of 1.6 to 0.3. Tables 8.10, 8.11 and 8.12 show some of the results.

Bailey (1974) showed that the available lysine content of maize fell from 95% in untreated grain to 22% in a toasted breakfast cereal [749a].

While it is evident that some processes can severely reduce the protein quality of cereals it is necessary to consider the foods in perspective. Since they are almost invariably consumed together with milk, cereal-plus-milk must be considered as the food in question. (This principle has been accepted by the U.S. Authorities since they permit packets of breakfast cereals to list both the nutrients in the cereal and in the cereal-plus-milk.) The protein values of cereal-plus-milk were examined by Womack *et al.*

TABLE 8.11. Heat damage to oat preparations (from Stewart *et al.*, 1943 [294])

	Protein efficiency ratio
Drum dried (boiled 15 min, dried 15 s, 130°C)	1.6
Rolled oats	1.5
Oven exploded (cooked 1–2 min at 100 lb, dried 1–2 min at 200°C)	1.6
Preparation of 75% oat, 20% corn and rye (boiled, dried, heated 80–100 lb, 190–232°C for 52–62 min, exploded)	0.5
Puffed oats (heated 5 min, 122°C, then live steam 200 lb, 198°C, 2 min, and then puffed)	0.3

TABLE 8.12. Nutritive value of breakfast cereals assayed on man (Murlin *et al.*, 1938 [276])

	Egg replacement value*
Pre-cooked oats	77
Granulated wheat and wheat germ	73
Wheat endosperm	85
Torn wheat	66
Flaked wheat	73
Toasted whole wheat	66
Inflated wheat	69

* Comparison of N balance on test diet and egg diet.

(1974) [305]; eleven cereal products ranging in protein content from 6% (puffed rice) to 15% (instant oatmeal and puffed wheat) mixed with 4 parts of liquid milk (dried skim milk powder was used in the rat diets).

In three of the products the protein quality of the mixture was higher than that of the milk alone; in five products there was no difference; in another three the protein quality was lower than that of milk alone. These three had been subjected to the most severe heat treatment, namely puffed rice, puffed wheat and high-protein flakes.

This is still not the complete assessment since apart from effects on the quality the addition of cereal to the milk increases the total quantity of protein consumed. The increase ranged from 33% to 120% for the different products. Finally, it is necessary to put the protein consumed in this dish into context of the whole day's food – the cereal-milk dish provided between 4 and 8 g of protein.

More recently high-temperature short-time treatment of wheat has been developed to produce the desired toasted product without damage to the protein and little loss of thiamin [275]. Conventional processing leaving the moisture content at 20% did not damage the protein and destroyed 25% of the thiamin. More severe treatment leaving the moisture level at 10% destroyed 70% of the thiamin. The same type of product was achieved by HTST treatment 230°C for 15 s leaving 10% moisture and destroying 35% of the thiamin. When the treatment was continued for 40 s the thiamin loss became 80% and PER fell from 1.3 to 0.9.

FRUITS AND VEGETABLES

Vitamin C is by far the most important nutrient in fruits and vegetables so most of the work has been concerned with this vitamin. As described in the section on vitamin C, destruction can occur during even short storage of fresh unprocessed fruits and vegetables through oxidation by internal oxidases initiated by cell damage. This occurs during wilting, which particularly affects leafy vegetables (and is reduced to some extent under cool, humid conditions), and also by bruising, which almost inevitably accompanies mechanical harvesting and handling. Fafunso and Bassir (1976) [330] showed that leaves lost 5–18% of their vitamin C only 2 h after picking, rising to 10–30% after 4 h, 35–60% after 8 h, and 38–66% after 10 h – the time at which they were purchased in that locality – finally, up to 90% was lost after 24 h.

Foods differ in the extent of their losses, for example tomatoes do not appear to lose vitamin C after severe bruising or even slicing yet the juice itself can lose the vitamin very rapidly – as much as 95% loss in 2 min [355].

Legumes can lose vitamin C on storage. For example Lima (butter) beans showed a loss of 40% of the vitamin C after 48 h at room temperature and 70% after 96 h. When removed from the pod the loss was 70% in 48 h. Cooling reduces, but does not prevent, this loss. After 48 h in the refrigerator loss was 5% and after 96 h, 20%. Beans removed from the pod lost 16% in 48 h in the refrigerator [415].

McCoombs (1957) showed that losses depended (to some extent) on the amount of oxidases present in the food. For example, after 4-6 days storage at 13°C and 75–80% RH there was no loss from kohlrabi and chard, 10% was lost from cabbage, 30% from kale, 20–40% from collards (depending on the season of harvest) and 40–50% from squash. The greatest losses were found in foods with the greatest amounts of oxidases [361].

Cell damage can take place at low temperatures through the formation of ice crystals, as described on p. 46, so that the temperature of storage is critical. Zepplin and Elvehjem (1944) showed that lettuce and broccoli stored in crushed ice lost 10% of the vitamin C in 3 days compared with 30% when stored in a wire basket in the refrigerator [664].

Processing losses obviously depend on the conditions and can vary up to 100%. Standard textbooks suggest that, in the absence of precise information of processing, cooking and handling it is advisable to assume a loss of 50% from vegetables. Good practice can reduce this to 25%. The average loss in hospital cooking was shown to be 75% [917].

Steaming caused a loss of 15–20% from kohlrabi, Brussels sprouts, cauliflower and potatoes; braising caused a loss of 30%. Beans lost more than the other vegetables, figures being 25–35% and 40–50% respectively for the two methods of cooking [342].

Heat sterilisation led to losses of 20–50% from spinach, 0–23% from peas and 20–35% from beans [920].

Bender et al. (1977) [313a] found enormous differences between foods cooked in different school kitchens on different occasions – vitamin C in cabbage ranged between 1.3 and 20 mg per 100 g. This means that the average allowance of 50% is a very crude approximation and direct analysis is almost always essential.

Several points arise. First, some foods are more susceptible to loss than others. Secondly, the total amount is important rather than the proportion lost. For example, a Malaysian dish, Acar, consisting of tomatoes, cucumber, carrots and chillies tossed in vinegar and spices showed only 40% loss from the fresh state to the plate, but this figure was derived from an initial content of 18 and a final content of 11 mg/100 g; on the other hand spring greens, which lost 50% in the cooking, still supplied 40 mg/100 g of cooked food.

This illustrates the third point, namely, that while it is usual to laud raw compared with cooked vegetables as a source of vitamin C, they are not necessarily superior, since more of the food may be consumed after cooking.

Abrams (1975) [308] illustrated some of the difficulties of attempting to generalise. When Brussels sprouts were cooked for 10 min, 28% of the vitamin C was lost, rising after 20 min to 36%. Palatability required a cooking time of 20 min. However, if deep cross-cuts were made in the butts of the sprouts the cooking time was reduced to 10 min and more of the vitamin was conserved.

Apart from vitamin C several fruits and vegetables are valuable sources of carotene, and to a lesser extent, other nutrients. Clearly, water-soluble nutrients are at greater risk than fat-soluble materials. Some representative results were provided by Olliver, 1967 [730] – Table 8.13 – and Weits *et al.*, 1970 [390] – Table 8.14.

TABLE 8.13. Ascorbic acid losses in vegetables during household cooking (after Olliver, 1967 [730])

Method	Vitamin C (%)		
	Destroyed	Extracted	Retained
Green vegetables			
Boiling (long time, much water)	10–15	45–60	25–45
Boiling (short time, little water)	10–15	15–30	55–75
Steaming	30–40	<10	60–70
Pressure cooking	20–40	<10	60–80
Root vegetables (*unsliced*)			
Boiling	10–20	15–25	55–75
Steaming	30–50	<10	50–70
Pressure cooking	45–55	<10	45–55

TABLE 8.14. Representative losses from cooked foods (Weits *et al.*, 1970 [390])

Nutrient	Spinach	Peas	Green beans
Vitamin C	65	30	20
Vitamin B_1	40	10	0
Vitamin B_2	30	20	10
Carotene	15	5	10
Iron	85	10	0
Potassium	35	20	10
Calcium	10	5	0

Trimming losses

There is an inevitable loss of nutrients when parts of the food are discarded, but since the distribution of nutrients in most fruits and vegetables is not uniform, losses of nutrients are not always proportional to the weight of the waste [674].

For example, the peel of apples and pears has 5–10 times as much vitamin C as the flesh and a higher proportion of the niacin, folate and riboflavin. Citrus fruits have proportionately more vitamin C in the peel, which except in the preparation of marmalade is discarded. Tomatoes have a greater concentration of riboflavin, niacin and vitamin C in the skin so affecting the relative amounts found in peeled products or in the juice (Table 1.5), p. 10.

The outer leaves of lettuce and cabbage, which are usually discarded, contain more carotene than inner leaves; there is more thiamin in the heart of cabbage than in outer leaves but the riboflavin is evenly distributed. Reports of the distribution of vitamin C in cabbage and lettuce differ, possibly because the proportions of outer green to white leaves vary with growing conditions and also because the outer leaves wilt before the inner leaves with consequent destruction of the vitamin C.

The outer parts of carrots, which are likely to be removed by machine peeling, are richer in carotene, thiamin, riboflavin and niacin. Spinach stems, on the contrary, which are the parts most likely to be discarded, have less vitamin C than the leaves.

Fruit juices

Fruit juices are mainly, almost only, of nutritional value because of their vitamin C content, so most of the work has been devoted to this aspect and a great deal of it has involved orange juice.

Much of the processing of fruit juices involves heating, for concentration, sterilisation or at least pasteurisation, but little if any damage is caused since vitamin C is relatively stable in acid solution. Even boiling orange juice in an open pan for 10 min destroyed only 10% [352]. There was no loss through drying under vacuum or foam-mat drying first to a five-fold concentration, and finally to a dry powder. The dried material was stable so long as the moisture content was kept down to 1%.

Horowitz et al. (1976) [347] examined the vitamin C content of a small number of samples of pasteurised and frozen orange juice preparations since they regarded these as new products compared with canned juices which have been extensively studied. This was not a controlled examination of the effects of processing. Four samples of fresh juice contained 67–70 mg/100 g ascorbic acid, 3–8 mg dehydroascorbic acid and 4–7 mg of inactive diketogulonic acid. Three samples of frozen juice were similar but six samples of pasteurised juice had less vitamin C – 38–59 mg AA and 1–4 mg DHA with correspondingly more diketogulonic acid, namely 15–30 mg. Since fresh juice lost no vitamin C on heating to 77°C with stirring these authors suggest that the loss during pasteurisation was not due to heat and air alone. They found 10% loss when frozen juice was diluted with tap water and stored for 7 days and suggested that metals in the water may be partly responsible.

Storage losses are almost entirely due to oxidation and are very small if oxygen is excluded (see also p. 46). There is some chemical destruction, including darkening of the colour, which is increased at higher temperatures. Such damage is greater in concentrates than in dilute juices because of the higher concentration of sugars, acids and nitrogenous compounds that facilitate the chemical reactions. For this reason even canned products are preferably stored under cool conditions. At 4°C there was no difference between single strength juices and concentrates, but at 49°C there was a marked difference and the rate of deterioration was related to temperature. Kefford (1973) [352] recommended storage at 10°C, when both hot-packed and aseptically sealed glass bottles lost only 1% of their vitamin C per month. At 18°C losses were only 5–10% in one year and 10–20% after two years. At subtropical temperatures of 24°C losses were 25% after 1 year and 50% after two years.

The air left in the headspace of cans and bottles causes rapid loss of vitamin C, but after the oxygen has been used the vitamin can be stable for long periods. Adam (1941) [309] showed greater stability in unlacquered tinned cans because the oxygen was rapidly removed by electrochemical corrosion. Where there is access of air, even the very slow diffusion through the walls of plastic containers, then destruction is continuous.

Orange juice stored in waxed cartons at 5°C lost 5–7% of the vitamin C per week, and up to 8% in larger containers because of the greater opportunity for oxidation [376]. Berry et al. (1971) reported a loss of 45% of the vitamin C from orange juice kept in paper cartons compared with 30% in plastic bottles [314].

Bender (1958) [313] found that bottled 'orange squash' (concentrated juice plus acid, flavour and sugar) lost a small amount of vitamin C initially due to the oxygen in the headspace, with no further loss after 6 months at ambient temperatures, 20% loss after 12 months and 60% loss after 2 years. These losses did not appear to be affected by exposure to light. The main cause of destruction is oxygen, since once the bottles were opened the loss of vitamin C was 10–20% in 8 days and 80–95% in 40 days at room temperatures (Table 3.6). This finding serves to illustrate the discrepancy between the nutritional value of a food when manufactured or even when purchased compared with that of the food when it is consumed.

Fruit juices are marketed in a considerable variety of containers made of different materials and in various sizes. Bissett and Berry (1975) [316] examined a range of these for the stability of the vitamin C in orange juice. Single-strength juice in tin-lined cans or glass bottles lost no vitamin C after 1 year storage at −18°C, 20% after 6 months at 27°C and 25% after 1 year at the same temperature.

Seven oz glass bottles were aseptically filled and stored for 1 year; losses were 13% at 4.4°C, 16% at 10°C and 21% at 15.6°C; when stored at 27°C, 30% was lost after 6 months.

Sixty-four oz polythene containers are permeable to air and even at −7°C the losses were 18% after 6 months; at 1°C the colour and flavour became unacceptable after 6 months and 62% of the vitamin C was destroyed.

Small, 4 oz, polystyrene containers were even worse because they are thinner but they are designed for rapid use after a very short storage period. After 1 week at temperatures up to 10°C the loss was 10% and this is apparently acceptable taking their low cost into consideration. However, even at −7°C there was 20% loss after 6 weeks, at 1°C the loss was 80% in this time – in marked contrast with the relatively high stability in glass and metal containers.

Large, 64 oz, cardboard containers were also poor, losses reached 75% after 3 weeks at 10°C: even at −7°C 20% of the vitamin was destroyed in 6 weeks, which was the same loss as in the polystyrene.

Alternative containers made from fibre lined with aluminium foil or with polythene both showed a loss of 10% in 1 year at −20°C. At −7°C, however, the foil barrier was better, the loss in 8 months being 20% compared with 60% from the polythene lined containers.

Frozen storage provides the best conditions, and Kefford (1973) [352] found no loss of vitamins C, B$_6$, biotin and folic acid after 8 months although Bissett and Berry (1975) found 10% loss of vitamin C in 1 year at 4°C regardless of headspace or preliminary treatment [316].

There is, as with all processing changes, a considerable difference between what is known from laboratory experimentation and what is achieved in commercial practice. Pelletier and Morrison (1965) [374] reported so great a lability of vitamin C in a number of orange-flavoured drinks that they stated that many fruit drinks on the market in Canada are unsatisfactory and not under proper control. Thirteen out of 20 liquid preparations were below label potency and the vitamin content fell rapidly when they were opened. The authors concluded that the fruit-flavoured drinks were either low in vitamin content when manufactured or subjected to excessively long storage periods. Pineapple juice was found to be up to 55 months in the distribution channels, with consequent vitamin loss [322].

Apple juice

The vitamin C concentration of apple juice is low and so not usually an important factor, but it also suffers from extreme instability. Even freeze-concentration (where the material is never subjected to heat) destroys the vitamin C.

PULSES AND OILSEEDS

These undergo similar changes in processing as well as having similar uses as sources of oil, of protein for both human and animal foods, and as raw materials in manufacture; and so they can be discussed together.

Legumes in particular, but also some of the oilseeds, provide examples of the beneficial effects of processing, since most of the 'antiphysiological factors' such as trypsin and amylase inhibitors, haemagglutinins, goitrogens and cyanogenic glycosides are destroyed by heat [409].

TABLE 8.15. Effect of home-cooking of bean preparations in Guatemala (Bressani, 1972 [408])

Product	PER	Available lysine (g/16 g N)	Protein (%)	Fat (%)	Crude fibre (%)
Raw beans	0	5.83	24.6	1.9	4.6
Cooked	1.24	6.30	24.9	0.7	2.8
Strained	1.43	6.35	24.0	0.6	1.6
Fried	0.87	5.17	17.8	13.3	1.6

Some of the pulses become harder during storage and their digestibility falls, accompanied by an increase in the amount of lignified protein; this can be prevented by heat. Pulses take a long time to cook and their digestibility is as low as 70–80%, so there is a great deal of interest in pre-treatment and instantisation processes (p. 117).

Oilseed meals are a byproduct of the vegetable oil industry and for many years there was little interest in processing damage to the protein residue. More recently the optimal processing conditions have been thoroughly investigated, particularly since they can be used for human food.

The main processing problem in both pulses and oilseeds is that of destroying the toxins without, at the same time, damaging the protein. Cottonseed, for example, contains gossypol which can combine with lysine so lowering the nutritive value of the protein as well as being directly toxic [765]. It can be destroyed if the meal is properly heated [414] as originally shown by Osborne and Mendel in 1917, but an alternative is to breed strains of cottonseed free from the toxin.

The toxins often depress the nutritive value of the protein. For example, Onayemi and Potter (1976) [452] prepared cowpeas by soaking, dehulling, grinding, supplementing with methionine and finally drum drying. The Protein Efficiency Ratio increased from 1.3 to 1.6 on drying. Storage for 24 weeks at 37°C resulted in a fall in PER, but not at 30°C. See also Table 8.15.

An additional problem arises when the oil is extracted with solvent since there can be a reaction with the protein to form toxic compounds. For example, ethylene dichloride can combine with cysteine in the protein and the product is toxic to calves, as discussed under Proteins, p. 72 [806].

Groundnuts *Arachis hypogaea*

Groundnuts contain trypsin inhibitors and there is an increase in protein utilisation on heating, followed by a decrease on overheating. Table 8.16

TABLE 8.16. Effect of heat on protein quality of groundnuts (Neucere *et al.*, 1972 [450])

Groundnuts	(°C)	PER	ALV
Raw		1.4	1.95
Wet heat	110	1.8	3.08
	120	1.5	2.78
	130	1.5	2.40
	145	1.3	2.03
	155	1.1	2.03
Dry heat	110	1.5	2.48
	120	1.9	3.08
	130	1.6	2.63
	140	1.2	2.33
	155	1.0	2.18

shows the relation between heat treatment and PER and available lysine [450]. Since groundnut protein is limited by the sulphur amino acids, processing damage restricted to available lysine can occur without showing as a fall in PER. Neucere *et al.* (1972) showed that there was no trypsin inhibitor remaining after moist heat at 110°C but there was some still remaining after dry heat at 130°C, under which conditions the PER was reduced. On this basis there does not appear to be a correlation between nutritional damage and trypsin inhibitor activity [450].

Anantharaman and Carpenter (1969) [397] showed that moist and dry heat at 121°C for 0.5 h were accompanied by a small and statistically non-significant rise in NPU from 0.40 to 0.43. Dry heat at 121°C for 4 h caused a fall in NPU to 0.28 due to a reduction in available lysine – there was no loss of available methionine.

Roasting is the commonest process to which groundnuts for human consumption are exposed and the protein is damaged, since temperatures are higher than those used by Anantharaman and Carpenter (1969), above. For example heating at 180°C for 25 min reduced NPU from 0.44 to 0.20. In the presence of moisture the NPU was 0.30, and in both instances damage was limited to lysine, both total and available [474].

Thiamin is largely destroyed during roasting – over 90% was destroyed in 20 min at 155-160°C [419].

In the Orient defatted groundnuts are treated by steaming and then inoculating with a fungus (*Neurospora* or *Rhizopus*). The fermentation leads to an increase in thiamin of up to 60%, varying in amount with the type of mould; riboflavin increases up to 300%; niacin up to 70%; there was no change in pantothenate [455]. Protein quality was not affected by fermentation. See also p. 115.

Soybeans

Soybeans constitute by far the largest crop of any of the pulses, and vast numbers of publications have been devoted to examining processing conditions since Osborne and Mendel first showed, in 1917, that raw soybeans would not support growth in rats.

Soybeans contain a variety of toxic factors, and since their destruction is accompanied by a fall in urease activity and in protein solubility, these can be used as an index of toxin destruction [437, 439]. The biological value of raw beans is about 0.6, rising to 0.7 as the toxins are destroyed and falling as the protein is damaged by further heating. Moisture facilitates heat penetration and so permits treatment at a lower temperature but involves heating a second time to dry the product. Hackler *et al.* (1965) [422] reported the following values which illustrate the relationships: (initial trypsin inhibitor content 14%).

Air inlet temp. (°C)	Retention of inhibitor (%)	PER
166	10	2.2
182	8	2.1
227	4	2.0
277	5	1.6
316	3	0.2

The authors compared the above figures with drum drying (150°C), vacuum drying (108°C) and freeze-drying, which all gave products with PER 2.2.

Protein damage in general is discussed in chapter 4. In soya, cystine is the first amino acid to be damaged, and the presence of reducing sugars enhances the effect on this and other amino acids. When mixed with other foods as a protein supplement it suffers more damage than when it is heated alone, in the same way as meat is more sensitive when mixed with other foods (p. 125). For example, a sample of drum-dried full fat soya had PER 2.1, NPU 0.46. When it had been dried with added banana to prepare a weaning food the PER was only 1.4, NPU 0.33. The damage was to the S-amino acids since the addition of methionine increased the PER to 2.2 [468].

Badenhop and Hackler (1971) [401] examined the effects of dry roasting (as commonly used for coffee, cocoa and peanuts) and showed that optimum palatability is gained at the expense of nutritional value. Four minutes roasting at 170°C produced the highest PER, namely 1.7, whereas the most palatable product had been roasted at 180°C, when PER fell to 1.46; at 185°C it fell to 1.28. (These results may not be completely reliable since the experimental animals ate slightly less of the more strongly heated food and this alone would reduce PER.)

At 180°C the fall in PER was accompanied by the following amino acid losses; tryptophan 35%, total lysine 17%, available lysine 31%, cystine 15% (no loss of methionine) and histidine 6%.

Hutton and Thompson (1975) treated soybeans by the micronisation process (infrared heat) and showed an increase in BV from 0.53 to 0.76 [617]. Wing and Alexander (1971) [663] showed that microwave heating caused less damage than dry heat. Peanuts behave in a similar fashion [450]. The effects of extrusion are discussed separately, p. 118.

Commercial production

There is, unfortunately, a discrepancy between the knowledge of the factors controlling the optimal processing conditions and their practical application in the factory, as illustrated by a series of samples purchased in the open market in the United States [441]. The Protein efficiency ratio of three concentrates ranged between 0.3 and 1.9, compared with value of 2.2 referred to above. On further heating they all improved to 2.1, indicating insufficient processing. Four samples of isolated soya protein ranged between 1.4 and 1.8; all except one improved to 2.0 on further heating, the remaining sample at PER 1.5 had been overheated.

Enrichment with methionine

It has been suggested that soya products, particularly those intended to replace meat, should be enriched with methionine – as is already done with some brands – to improve their nutritional value. Shemer and Perkins (1975) [467], however, showed that added methionine is more sensitive to heat damage than methionine in protein combination – 30% of the latter was lost by heating for 1 h, while all the added methionine was destroyed.

There is an additional problem of the potential toxicity of added methionine and the unpleasant flavour of at least some samples of synthetic methionine.

Garden peas (*Pisum sativum*)

These are an important crop in many countries – providing protein, vitamin C and thiamin, their relative importance in the diet obviously depending on the amount eaten, the remainder of the diet and processing damage. Their processing has been extensively studied, particularly losses of vitamin C, and they serve to illustrate many of the problems involved.

Peas are eaten in the fresh green state or processed by drying, canning and freezing, as well as being left to mature on the plant.

Robertson and Sissons (1966) [462] showed that the loss of vitamin C varied with variety and that the content decreased during maturation and also during 5 days storage. At the same time cooking losses increased – peas stored for 1 day lost 10% into the cooking water compared with 30% after 5 days storage, while loss by oxidation increased from 7% to 30%. Another more detailed example of the varietal differences is given in chapter 1 [442].

The proper assessment of nutritional changes in processing is a comparison of the fresh and processed foods after cooking, i.e. when consumed rather than a comparison before and after processing, and peas were used to illustrate this point earlier (Tables 1.1 and 1.2). Freezing and freeze-drying do destroy some of the vitamin C, but after the shorter cooking time that the treated food requires the processed foods are not inferior to fresh peas [462].

Freezing caused a loss of 25–30%; subsequent cooking in a small volume of water caused a loss of 35–45%; the final product contained *12–16 mg/100 g.*

Accelerated freeze-drying caused a loss of 20–30%; subsequent cooking, 30–40%; final product contained *13–18 mg.*

Air drying cost 30–40%; cooking in the larger volume of water needed cost 50–60%; final product contained *11–12 mg.*

Canning cost 50–60%; reheating cost 5% (0–20%); final product contained *8–11 mg.*

Fresh peas cooked for 10 min 1–5 days after harvesting contained 16–19 mg vitamin C/100 g which is within the same range as frozen and freeze-dried cooked peas.

Samples harvested on 12 successive days [446] showed that maturation reduced the vitamin C from 220 mg/100 g dry weight to 120 mg, but there was no effect on thiamin content (1.6–1.7 mg/100 g dry weight). As the peas matured there was a fall in the ratio of skin to cotyledons, and there is twice as much vitamin C in the skin.

Vitamin C can be destroyed when a food is mechanically damaged, since it is then brought into contact with the oxidase. When pods of peas were opened by hand there was no loss of the vitamin in 120 min, but after machine podding there was a steady loss totalling 10% over this period. Similarly, vining on a commercial scale destroyed 15% more of the vitamin C than vining on a miniature scale [446].

The effects of blanching at 96–98°C for 1 min followed by cooling in a water spray for 6 s depended on the variety of pea. One variety lost 10% of the vitamin C, four lost 20% and a sixth variety lost 30%. Thiamin was more stable, two varieties showed no loss, two showed 10% loss, one showed 20% loss, and the variety (Scout) that showed the greatest loss of vitamin C, namely 30%, lost 40% of its thiamin.

The overall process took about 90 min, from initial washing, through blanching, cooling first in water then in air, and finally freezing, and the only significant loss was at the blanching stage. There was no loss during freezing. The final measurement, the one that matters to the consumer, was the vitamin C content after cooking. Fresh peas were boiled for 6.3 min, plus 1.1 min taken to bring the water to the boil, and lost 40% of their vitamin C. Frozen peas were boiled for 3 min, plus 3 min taken to bring them to the boil. The overall processing cost of 11% of the vitamin C plus 30% in the final cooking – the total loss being the same as that of fresh peas.

POTATOES

Potatoes are an important source of energy and protein in some parts of the world, but even in many industrialised countries they supply a large proportion of the vitamins C and B_1. Processing losses can, therefore, be a serious matter.

The vitamin content varies considerably with the variety and growing conditions – vitamin C can range between 1.1 and 55 mg/100 g [479]; in a series of 147 samples niacin ranged between 1.03 and 2.08 mg/100 g and vitamin B_6 between 0.13 and 0.42 mg/100 g [493, 477].

Losses of nutrients can take place: 1. during storage of the tubers after harvesting – a period that may extend over many months, 2. in peeling and cooking, 3. during processing, which involves peeling and cooking and may be followed by drying or canning and 4. by oxidation when kept hot before consumption.

There is a problem in attempting to ascertain losses because all 'before' and 'after' analyses are necessarily carried out on different tubers and there can be as much variation between individual potatoes in control groups as between treated and controls so that some of the observations are uncertain [500].

Storage

Storage of the tubers particularly affects vitamin C, which is lost at the rate of about 10% per month, depending on variety, temperature and humidity. Augustin *et al.* (1975) [478] showed that the rate of loss of vitamin C was linear with the logarithm of time at 7°C and 95% RH.

As an average value, under commercial conditions potatoes initially contain about 30 mg vitamin C/100 g and finish 7–8 months later with about 10 mg [909, 479] – Table 8.17.

TABLE 8.17. Vitamin C in fresh and processed potatoes $\pm$ S.E. (Bring *et al.*, 1963 [479])

	mg/100 g wet wt Peeled raw[1]	Loss (%) Boiled mashed[2]	Dried flakes[3]
October 1960	29.3±0.7	22.2±2.4	56.9±1.2
February 1961	11.7±0.2	22.9±2.4	63.5±1.1
May 1961	10.6±0.2	24.9±3.1	61.7±1.2

[1] Russet Burbanks stored 3°C January, February to 12°C in May.
[2] Boiled 25–30°C.
[3] Analysed after reconstituting with hot water but calculated to dry weight basis.

Niacin and riboflavin are maintained but thiamin appears to fluctuate, possibly due to sprouting [493, 478]. Vitamin B_6 increased steadily during storage, in one variety by 90% and in another by 150%. This was attributed to the liberation of bound forms of the vitamin.

Preparation

As much as 40% of the total material can be discarded in peeling, depending on the method – hand-peeling, machine-peeling or lye-peeling. Subsequent soaking in water, which in some catering institutions can occupy 14 to 24 h, leaches out considerable amounts of the vitamin C and B_1, despite the small surface-to-volume ratio. Zarnegar and Bender (1971) [500] found 10–20% loss of vitamin C on soaking peeled whole potatoes overnight, irrespective of whether they had been peeled by hand or machine; Eddy and Stock (1972) [482] found 20% loss after hand-peeling and 30% loss after machine-peeling. On the other hand long soaking in oxygenated water can result in the synthesis of vitamin C [482].

Most of the reported investigations involve vitamin C; much less work has been done on the losses of thiamin, which are enhanced by the addition of sulphite used to prevent discolouration. Oguntona and Bender (1976) [492] showed that thiamin can be leached out of the deeper layers and that losses from a layer 10 mm from the cut surface were 20% in tap water and 55% in sulphite solution. On subsequent frying there was a further loss of 10%, which was doubled in the samples that had been soaked in sulphite.

In commercial practice the potatoes, whole or chipped, are immersed in sulphite solution, drained and then stored for varying periods. Mapson and Wager (1961) [488a] showed that it was possible to store potatoes for 7 days at 5°C and 14 days at 1°C; losses of thiamin reached 24% after 3 days storage at 5°C. Subsequent boiling brought about an additional loss of 15% in the absence of sulphite and 30% after sulphiting; frying destroyed 10% in non-sulphited potatoes but this increased to 35–45% loss after sulphiting.

Cooking

The greater loss of vitamin C is by leaching into the cooking water, and there is little true destruction. The extent of losses of vitamin C and some of the variables are illustrated by a series of analyses by Domah *et al.* (1974) [481]. Slices 3–6 mm thick were cooked under various conditions: unpeeled in distilled water, 10% loss; after peeling the loss was 45%. Boiling in saline caused a greater loss than in distilled water – 15 mg/100 g was left after boiling in saline compared with 26 mg in salt-free water. Frying caused only small losses, since the high temperature tends to seal up the surface and protects the vitamin C; only 18% was lost after frying for 30 min at 140°C. Examples are given in Tables 8.17 and 8.18.

As mentioned above under Preparation, there is some destruction of thiamin on boiling and frying – 10–15% – which is greatly increased when the potatoes have been treated with sulphite – 20–45%.

Food Composition Tables [909] provide average figures for losses of vitamin C from the raw state to eventual consumption as follows: 20–50% on boiling peeled potatoes, 20–40% on deep frying, but values in practice vary enormously.

The greatest destruction by far is by oxidation when the food is kept hot after cooking and this time can obviously range from zero to an hour or more. Bender *et al.* (1977) [313a] found very large differences in total vitamin C content between potatoes cooked in different school kitchens on different occasions. For example the vitamin C in boiled, mashed potatoes ranged between zero and 6.5 mg and in roast potatoes ranged between 0.8 and 18.9 mg/100 g. The main cause of these large differences is probably the length of time the food was kept hot. Table 8.18 shows the rapid loss of vitamin C – 33% in 0.5 h increasing to 60% in 3 h – when mashed potatoes are kept hot.

Other vitamins are much more stable than the vitamin C. Page and Hanning (1963) [493] found 5% loss of niacin and 10% of vitamin B_6 on

TABLE 8.18. Loss of vitamins in mashed potatoes subject to various heat treatments (instant potato flakes plus skim milk and margarine) (Ang *et al.*, 1975 [574])

	°C*	C	B_2	B_1
Freshly prepared	63	0	0	0
held 0.5 h	66	33	0	0
1.5 h	74	50	0	10
3.0 h	79	60	0	20
Frozen mashed potato (to simulate convenience food system handling)				
Frozen-thawed	7	0	0	
Frozen, reheated in convection oven and held 0.5 h	65	0	10	
ditto: infrared oven	75	5	10	
ditto: steamer	60	5	15	
ditto: microwave oven	75	5	10	

* Maximum temperature during holding.

baking, with 20% loss of niacin and 10% of B_6 on boiling, most of this being extracted into the water. Similarly when potatoes are kept hot after cooking thiamin is far more stable than vitamin C and riboflavin is completely stable, Table 8.18. Reheating of frozen potato led to considerable loss of vitamin C but little loss of riboflavin and niacin [574].

Processing

Potatoes are subjected to a wide variety of processes ranging from dehydration to partial or complete pre-cooking or canning, and may be treated with sulphite, which destroys the thiamin.

Myers and Roehm (1963) [491] examined a number of processed products and the great differences between samples indicates the losses. Two brands of diced potato contained, on dry weight basis, 9 and 20 mg vitamin C/100 g respectively and both lost 35% when cooked. Two brands of flakes contained 4.5 and 13 mg and lost 48% and 10% respectively on 'cooking'. Two brands of sliced potatoes contained 10 and 26 mg and lost 75% and 68% respectively on cooking.

These authors measured only reduced ascorbic acid since vitamin C is present almost wholly in this form in raw potatoes, but they offered no evidence whether this was still true after processing.

Somogyi *et al.* (1971) found little difference between home-prepared and factory processed chipped potatoes, potato crisps, mashed and canned and peeled potatoes [494].

TABLE 8.19. Vitamin C losses during production of dehydrated mashed potatoes (after Jadhav *et al.*, 1975 [488])

Add-back process		Freeze-thaw process	
Processing step	Loss (%)	Processing step	Loss (%)
Raw potatoes	0	Raw potatoes	0
Slicing and washing	9.3	Slicing	8.2
Blanching	16.9	Washing	14.5
Steam cooking	20.3	Steam cooking	17.4
Mashing (20 min, 60°C)	57.4	Mashing (2 min, 80°C)	17.6
Conditioning (cold air)	78.3	Freezing-thawing	16.2
Air lift drying	63.6*	Pre-drying	29.7
Fluid bed drying	58.4*	Granulation (fluid bed)	19.7*
Fluid bed cooling	57.0*	Final drying (10 min, 60°C)	18.9*

* Apparent increase attributed to the production of substances that interfere with the analysis

Canned potatoes lose soluble materials into the water or brine, which is usually discarded, and these losses will vary with the size of the potatoes and the storage time. Witkowski and Paradowski (1976) stated that one third of the vitamin C passed into the brine during the sterilisation alone, and that only 5–10% was destroyed [499].

Dehydration can result in complete destruction of vitamin C and thiamin, depending on the methods used. Cording *et al.* (1961) [480] destroyed 30% of the vitamin C by roller drying, with a further loss of 30% during 28 weeks storage of the dried flakes at 24°C and 5% moisture. Added vitamin C was also lost even when antioxidant was included but was retained when the product was stored under nitrogen. Sulphur dioxide destroyed the thiamin, but added vitamin A and niacin were stable to both processing and storage.

Jadhav *et al.* (1975) [488], Table 8.19, showed the loss at various stages and the differences between methods of treatment. In the 'add-back' process there is longer exposure to air and heat than in the freeze-thaw process and nearly 80% of the vitamin C was lost before the final drying stage. The apparent increase of vitamin C in the dried product was attributed by the authors to the formation of substances that interfered with both the 2,4-dinitrophenylhydrazine and polarographic methods of analysis.

Sulphite is sometimes incorporated into various forms of dehydrated potatoes to preserve both the colour and vitamin C (e.g. U.S. Patents 3 800 047 and 3 027 264) and this is likely to destroy a great deal of the thiamin. While vitamin C can be restored, added thiamin would normally be destroyed by the sulphite, but U.S. Patent 3 343 970 describes a method of restoring thiamin and adding sulphite at separate stages.

EGGS

Eggs are rich in protein, vitamin A, thiamin and riboflavin but are not usually eaten in sufficient amounts to make a major contribution to the diet. One of their most important contributions is the vitamin D, since this is present in so few foods. The iron of egg presents a complex problem. Whereas eggs are rich in iron it is present in a phosphoprotein complex which not only makes it unavailable but reduces the availability of some of the iron present in the intestine from other foods. So the addition of iron to a food or a meal adds to the iron intake but reduces the total amount that is available.

Egg protein has BV 1.0 and so shares with human milk the distinction of being a perfect protein. It is used as an alternative to the 'ideal amino acid mixture' as a standard for comparing the chemical score of proteins.

The nutrient content is little altered by the method of production. There was no difference between the amounts of most nutrients in eggs produced by battery, deep litter and free range methods – protein, cholesterol, thiamin, riboflavin, niacin, pantothenic acid and retinol were the same. There were small differences in calcium (10% less in the battery system), iron (5% less in deep litter), folic acid and vitamin B_{12} (both about 40% less in the battery system) tocopherols (20% greater in deep litter). Fat content and the amounts of different types of fats were the same in all three [511].

Eggs can be stored at 0°C for 12 months without loss of niacin, biotin, or choline, 10% loss of riboflavin and pantothenate, 25% folate and 50% vitamin B_6. After 3 months there was no loss of riboflavin, pantothenate or folate but 20% loss of vitamin B_6 (Evans *et al.*, in Harris and Karmas, 1975 [894]).

The small amount (1.2%) of reducing sugars present in egg results in rapid deterioration of dried egg during storage – loss of solubility and beating power, lowering of pH, and browning accompanied by development of unpleasant flavours [509]. Removal of the glucose by fermentation with yeast or glucose oxidase allows storage without deterioration and this is now normal practice.

Spray drying does not damage the vitamins (A, D, thiamin, riboflavin, pantothenic acid and niacin were examined by Hauge and Zscheile, 1942; Klose *et al.*, 1943; Denton *et al.*, 1944 and Whitford *et al.*, 1951 [508, 510, 502 and 512]).

Losses can occur on subsequent storage (despite the removal of glucose) dependent on the temperature. All the above listed vitamins except A were stable for 9 months at 70°C; at 21°C there was 50% loss of thiamin, 10% loss of riboflavin, but no loss of pantothenic acid or niacin. The last two were completely stable even at 37°C after 9 months.

Vitamin A was less stable, and there was a steady deterioration even at −10°C – 10% loss after 1 month, 20% after 2 months, 40% after 3 months and 60% after 9 months; at higher temperatures the losses were greater.

De Groot (1963) showed no change in BV of an egg product (egg, skim milk and oil) on pasteurisation [533].

Section E

Addition of Nutrients

Chapter 9

FOOD ENRICHMENT

The addition of nutrients to foods can be classed under three headings. When nutrients are added to a legally defined standard level the term enrichment is used. Fortification is the addition of nutrients that were not present in the food before processing or only in small amounts. Finally, supplementation of snack foods designed so that they make a special contribution to the diet is termed nutrification. In practice the terms enrichment and fortification are often used interchangeably.

A fourth term, restoration, is self-explanatory, meaning the restoration of nutrients lost in processing, for example, to milled grain where nutrients have been lost in the discarded bran and germ.

Compulsory enrichment is sometimes a combination of restoration and nutrification. For example, in Great Britain white flour is enriched with thiamin, niacin and iron which are partial restorations (only partial since they do not fully restore processing losses), and also calcium, which, since it is present in only small amounts in the whole grain, must be categorised as nutrification. Similarly in the United States riboflavin, which is present to only a small extent in the wheat berry, is added to white flour.

So much for details of nomenclature. Enrichment is often used as a general term. There are two modes of practice, legal enactment as a public health measure and voluntary additions to proprietary foods.

The latter may be of considerable benefit to the consumer, as for example in baby and toddler foods, where the added nutrients often play a useful rôle; alternatively, nutrients may be simply added for sales appeal since the need is not evident. In many circumstances voluntary fortification is a combination of the two since the extra nutrients may be of some benefit, if only to ensure adequate intake even if there is no evidence of need. Regulations permitting such additions differ considerably in different countries, as discussed later, some authorities giving a completely free hand to the manufacturer, others being more restrictive or completely restrictive.

Public health enrichment

So far as public health measures are concerned the procedure should follow a logical progress, although, historically, this has not always occurred.

1. Demonstrate the need to enrich, 2. establish the best vehicle to carry the nutrients, 3. ensure that there is no detriment to palatability and acceptability and that the cost is acceptable, 4. technology, and, 5. legal enforcement.

Enrichment is often desirable in developing countries but cannot be carried out because one or more of these stages presents an obstacle.

1. Demonstration of need would probably be essential at the present time in any country despite what may have happened in the past since there is considerable cost involved.

Although enrichment of white bread in the United States followed reports of inadequate *intake* of thiamin in a large part of the population there were no signs of deficiency. So far as the addition of vitamin A to margarine was concerned there was no evidence even of inadequate intake. It was rather a moral point since the rationing of butter in Great Britain during the Second World War effectively deprived the consumers of part of their vitamin intake which would, perhaps, have had nutritional repercussions, so the enrichment was carried out without clearly demonstrating a need. The outbreak of xerophthalmia in Denmark in 1916, consequent upon the export of butter and its replacement with unenriched margarine, was the source of evidence.

In many developing countries the need is obvious.

2. The vehicle is clearly of fundamental importance since it must be a food commonly consumed, especially by the population groups in greatest need. It must be one of the cheapest foods which is eaten in greater quantity by the poorer people; those who eat relatively little of the cheaper staple foods must be consuming a more varied diet and so are probably already obtaining an adequate intake of nutrients.

3. Enrichment cannot be carried out unless the nutrient is compatible with the food, i.e. a fat-soluble vitamin could not be added to an aqueous medium, although this particular problem has been overcome by the availability of water-dispersible forms of the vitamins. There must obviously be no change in colour, flavour or texture. This militates, for example, against high level fortification with iron since this can form coloured complexes as well as promote oxidation. Any increase in price may jeopardise the scheme or, at least, the increase must be very small.

At the same time any danger of excessive sensitivity to additions, even by a small number of people, must be considered. Too high a level of iron enrichment will affect those suffering from haemochromatosis, iodine may cause thyrotoxicosis, vitamin D has given rise to idiopathic hypercalcaemia.

4. The technology has posed considerable problems in the past, such as how to blend very small amounts of vitamin mixtures with large volumes of materials of different density, or how to add amino acids, vitamins or

minerals to whole cereal grains. The solutions have required considerable efforts in food technology and even when the problems have been solved the application often presents a major obstacle to enrichment in developing countries. One of the greatest obstacles lies in the very large number of small-scale processing plants where it would not be possible to control the additions; when communities rely largely or solely on foods that they grow themselves then enrichment is not the solution to their nutritional problems.

5. Finally, it is little use passing regulations if they cannot be enforced. Enrichment by law requires a machinery for sampling foods, for analysing possibly large numbers of samples in many different areas of the country, and, finally, of enforcing a penalty in the courts. Much potential enrichment has foundered on this point in countries where the population would clearly have benefited from enrichment.

An example of these stages is provided by the enrichment experiment in the Philippines in 1948–50.

The need was obvious: in 1947 there were 24 000 deaths from beri-beri and the incidence of the disease was 150 per 100 000 of the population. A test area, the peninsula of Bataan, was selected since this was sufficiently isolated to keep food supplies separate from those of an adjacent control area. In the test area the incidence of beri-beri was 13%, with 164 deaths among a population of 98 000. The intake of thiamin was 0.7 mg per head per day which is about half the recommended daily intake. It was decided to enrich with thiamin, riboflavin, niacin and iron, increasing the thiamin intake to 2 mg per day.

The vehicle was also obvious since rice was the staple food. The first problem was the technological one of handling such a bulk of food in factories and the second problem was adding the supplement, which was a powder, to the whole grain. The first problem was overcome by enriching one two-hundredth part of the food to 200 times the required concentration, i.e. preparing a pre-mix, then diluting this with the untreated rice. The second problem was overcome by the technique of spraying a solution of the additives on to the grains and coating them with a film of the protein zein. The additives would thus be retained when the rice was washed and even cooked but would be released during digestion.

A final technical problem arose from the yellow colour of riboflavin. Since only one in 200 grains of rice was enriched the yellow grains appeared to be occasional discoloured ones and were picked out by the housewife and discarded. There was no solution to this technological problem other than omitting riboflavin from the nutrient mixture.

The experiment was highly successful; after one year the death rate had fallen by 64% in the test area compared with a rise of 2% in the control area.

After 21 months there were no deaths from the disease and the incidence had fallen by 89%.

The last point of legal enforcement defeated the project; it was not possible to pass and enforce central legislation to ensure that all rice was enriched. The only nutritional solution in such cases is to put an enriched product on the market and promote its sales in competition with other kinds.

Restoration

Restoration is the most widespread of the enrichment programmes and is applied to the white bread in many countries (Table 9.1); very few countries compel enrichment of rice. Even countries which do not permit the addition of nutrients to foods do allow restoration. As the table shows there is some variation in the number and amount of nutrients added because of national policies. There may, in addition, be proprietary cereal products with varying amounts of various nutrients.

In Great Britain and Canada the nutrients are added to the flour, so that all flour products are enriched. This means that the onus is on the flour miller not the baker. In Great Britain the law demands that white flour, mostly 70% extraction rate, should be enriched at the rate of 14 oz of *creta preparata* (treated calcium carbonate) to the 280 lb sack (the standard sack used in British bakeries) which is equivalent to about 90 mg calcium per 100 g bread, and not less than 1.65 mg iron per 100 g flour, 0.24 mg thiamin and 1.6 mg niacin. All flour other than wholemeal (100% extraction) must be enriched.

In the United States enriched flour must contain not less than 0.44 mg B_1, 0.26 mg B_2, 3.6 mg niacin and 2.9 mg iron per 100 g of the flour; calcium is not specified. Although the levels set for bread are related to the flour and the 1943 Order of the U.S. War Food Administration applied, at the time, to the bread, in practice it is the dough that is enriched by the baker.

The other food that is commonly enriched for public health reasons is margarine, as listed in Table 9.2. It will be observed that enrichment is mainly carried out in the developed countries and few of the developing countries do so, for the reasons outlined above.

Since the early days of the Philippines experiment the enrichment of whole grains has become more sophisticated. For example, the HLR-Rickus procedure for enriching rice involves spraying an acidified solution of thiamin, niacin and vitamin B_6 in sorbitol and, after drying, coating with zein-stearic acid in alcohol solution and finally coating with shellac.

As a separate layer, tocopherol acetate in isopropanol is sprayed on with intermittent treatment with calcium phosphate to prevent stickiness. A layer of shellac separates this from the next coating of vitamin A, folic acid and zinc oxide. Another layer of shellac protects the vitamins from the layer of ferric orthophosphate. The grain is finally treated with calcium phosphate to whiten it and finished with talc to provide translucence. Such enriched food is stable for periods up to 6 months except for 10% loss of vitamin A.

In the Wright procedure ethyl cellulose in acetone and shellac are used as coating agents and the vitamins are stable to cooking.

A different approach is to soak the scarified (scratched) grains in a solution of vitamins, and often lysine, to take up the required quantity and then to dilute the pre-mix with untreated grain.

TABLE 9.1. Enrichment of cereal products (per kg)

	Thiamin mg	Riboflavin mg	Niacin mg	Iron mg	Calcium mg
Australia	1.6	2.4	16	14.7	1000
Brazil[1]	4.5	2.5	—	30	1000
Canada	4.4–5.5	2.7–3.3	35–44	29–36	1100–1400
Chile[1]	6.3	1.3	13	13.3	1700
(Rice)	4.4–8.8	2.6–5.3	35–70	29–57	1100–1650
Congo					
(Dem Rep)	4–6	2.5–3.5	32–45	26–35	1000–1500
Costa Rica	4.4–5.5	2.6–3.3	35–44	29–36	1100–1400
Denmark[1]	5	5	—	30	5000
(Rye flour)[1]	—	—	—	30	10 000
Dominica	4.4–5.5	2.6–3.3	35–44	29–36	1100–1400
Germany	3–4	1.5–5.0	20	30	720–2000
Israel	—	2.5	—	—	—
Japan	5	3	—	—	1500
Nicaragua	1	1.4	15.7	13	500
Panama[1]	4.4	2.6	35	28.7	1100
Peru[1]	4.0	4.0	30	20	1000
Philippines[1]	4.4–5.5	2.6–3.3	35–44	29–36	1100–1400
Portugal	4.4–5.5	2.6–3.3	35–44	28–36	—
Puerto Rico[1]	4.2	2.4–2.5	30	26–36	1100
Sweden	2.6–4.0	1.2	23–40	30	—
Switzerland	2.8–4.2	1.7–2.5	29–44	18–26	—
United Kingdom[1]	2.4	—	16	16.5	1250
United States[2]					
White flour	4.4–5.5	2.6–3.3	35–44	29–36	1100–1400
Bread	2.4–4.0	1.6–3.5	22–33	18–28	660–1750
Corn meal	4.4–6.6	2.6–4.0	35–53	29–57	1100–1600
Rice	4.4–8.8	2.6–5.3	35–70	29–57	1100–2200
Pastas	8.8–11.0	3.7–4.8	60–75	29–36	1100–1400
USSR	2–4	4	10–30	—	—

[1] Legally enforced. (*Note:* Some of the information in this table is a compromise between conflicting reports.)
[2] Legal enforcement in 30 States (vitamin D also added 8–50 μg/kg).

Yet another alternative is to make an artificial cereal grain, which must not be distinguishable from the natural grains, from a mixture of the amino acids, vitamins and minerals required, and then to blend this into the bulk of the untreated grain.

The history of enrichment of flour in Great Britain illustrates some of the reasons why the logical stages may not be followed. In 1941 synthetic

TABLE 9.2. Enrichment of margarine (per kg)

	Vitamin A μg	Vitamin D μg
Australia	9000	100
Austria	6000	25
Belgium	6000	25
Brazil	4500–15000	12.5–50
Canada	10000	—
Chile	9000	25
Denmark	6000	15
Finland	6000	62–90
Germany	6000–9000	7–25
Greece	7500	37
India	7500	—
Israel	9000	75
Japan	6000–12000	—
Mexico	6000	50
Netherlands	6000	25
Norway	6000	62
Portugal	6000–10000	22–25
Sweden	9000	37
Switzerland	9000	75
South Africa	6000	25
Turkey	6000	25
United Kingdom	9000	70–90
United States	10000	110

thiamin became available on a large scale and it was decided to add this to the white flour of 70–72% extraction rate. Before this policy could be implemented large shipping losses of wheat reduced stocks to a dangerously low level and it was decided to raise the extraction rate to 85% as an economy measure. This made fortification unnecessary but raised the problem that the higher phytate content might reduce the availability of calcium especially as milk was in limited supply (iron and zinc were not thought of as a problem at that time). Consequently calcium was added in the form of calcium carbonate at the rate, first of 7 oz, then of 14 oz per 280 lb sack of flour. With so high an extraction rate iron and thiamin and niacin were not necessary and riboflavin did not present any problems. At various times the extraction rate fluctuated between 85% and 95%.

In 1952 when the controls on the milling of wheat were lifted there was a universal desire to return to the white loaf of 70% extraction rate and it was decided to enrich this with some of the nutrients up to the level of the 80% extraction flour that had apparently contributed towards general good health of the wartime years; so the post-war loaf, other than wholemeal, was enriched with iron, thiamin, niacin and calcium.

A recommendation of the Food Standards Committee in 1974 stated that there was no problem of niacin deficiency among the British population since this is made in the body from tryptophan, and so niacin could safely be omitted from the enrichment programme. Calcium was also considered to be unnecessary since there were adequate amounts from other foods but the Committee were impressed with the observation that coronary heart disease was less common in areas where the water supply was hard, i.e. richer in calcium, than in soft water areas, and until this has been explained the Committee thought it safer to continue to include calcium in the bread.

Voluntary enrichment

A wide variety of manufactured foods are voluntarily enriched. For example most, if not all, infant milk formulae contain a range of nutrients and most infant cereal products contain added thiamin, riboflavin and niacin, vitamin D, calcium and iron. Some include vitamin A and others have a complete range including B_6, B_{12}, folate and pantothenate.

Most breakfast cereals are enriched, some with a limited range of the vitamins and iron, others with a more complete range, sometimes including vitamin C and additional protein.

One of the earliest nutrients to be added to foods was iodine to prevent goitre. It was suggested as long ago as 1833 by Boussingault and adopted in Switzerland shortly after 1900, when it was added to chocolate. A commoner vehicle for iodine is salt (sodium chloride) but in most countries this is done only on a voluntary basis so that it is available in areas where it is needed rather than compulsorily provided for everyone since problems can arise from indiscriminate fortification with iodine.

Enrichment of milk with vitamin D was started in the United States in 1931 because of the common occurrence of rickets.

There are public health programmes covering a variety of staple foods in many countries but they are not legally enforced and so, although fostered by governments, they are voluntary. Enrichment programmes for rice have been developed in Colombia, Taiwan, Hawaii, Japan, United States and Venezuela. Maize is enriched in several states of the United States, Egypt,

Mexico and Yugoslavia. Margarine enrichment is mandatory in some countries and voluntary in others.

The amino acids lysine and methionine, one or other of which is limiting in almost every food and diet, are available on a large scale and are occasionally used to raise the biological value of the protein of a food. A paradox arises when lysine is added to cereal foods since, while the protein quality of that specific food is improved, diets as a whole are usually limited by the sulphur amino acids and so would not be improved by lysine. It is being used in some developing countries.

Some proprietary foods are enriched with protein although it could be argued that any country sufficiently technically developed to do this has no need for extra protein.

Regulations

Clearly any nutrient can be added to foods so long as it does not affect acceptability but there are regulations governing such additions in many countries.

The Food Law Research Centre in Brussels has suggested that enrichment is justified when processing leads to substantial losses and when the food in question constitutes an important source of the nutrient and cheaper substitutes would cause a gap in intake.

Great Britain is the only country where manufacturers may fortify their products with any nutrient without requiring permission. Claims may be made only for a limited number of nutrients but others may be added and listed on the package as ingredients. There is a voluntary Code of Practice in Advertising (which has not the force of law) stating that no claims should be made for vitamins unless an average portion of the food supplies at least one-sixth of the recommended intake (which is specified); that a food should not be claimed as a rich source unless it supplies one-half of the RDI, and not termed therapeutic unless it supplies the full RDI.

In France restoration is permitted to cereal foods to a level of 80–200% of the 'natural' levels, taking the highest level found in the four major cereal grains as the standard. There is a general fear of widespread indiscriminate fortification with possible imbalance of nutrients. Public opinion is against sophistication and fortification of foods as a general policy. Nothing is added to margarine and, apart from cereal restoration, only special dietetic foods may be enriched.

Similar arguments are advanced in Norway; iodine may be added to salt and vitamins to bread but little is done in practice. Iron is not yet added to flour but has been under discussion.

In Sweden restoration is permitted so long as the additions do not alter the nutritional profile, i.e. the balance of nutrients naturally present in the original foodstuff. Denmark is less restrictive following changes in 1973. Wheat flour is compulsorily enriched with 5 mg thiamin, 5 mg riboflavin, 30 mg iron and 5 g calcium carbonate per kg; oatmeal is widely consumed in Denmark and to overcome the rachitogenic effect, since 1935 1% calcium acid phosphate is mixed with the oatmeal during milling together with vitamin A at 4.2 mg/kg. Since the adult diet is rather rich in phosphate, calcium was added to wheat flour as carbonate, but for children it was considered desirable to retain the ratio by adding both calcium and phosphate, so in wheat groats, commonly eaten by children, it was decided to add calcium as phosphate.

Denmark was the first country to adopt enrichment of margarine in 1937. Retinol, carotene and vitamin D were added at the same level as in butter, and when improved feeding of cows raised the levels in butter, the amount in margarine was increased in 1952 to 4.2 mg retinol, 1 mg carotene and 12 μg vitamin D per kg – still below the enrichment level in many other countries. Since 1973 the regulations have been less restrictive and proprietary foods may be enriched, but only after demonstrating a need and obtaining permission.

In Holland, margarine is enriched, all salt is iodised (including that used in baking) and baby foods are enriched. Otherwise only restoration is allowed unless permission is obtained from the minister.

Belgian regulations date back to a law of 1853 forbidding the addition of anything to bread (to prevent adulteration) so only margarine and dietetic foods are enriched.

In Germany few foods are enriched. Enrichment of proprietary foods by manufacturers requires permission of the minister and such foods are marketed as dietetic foods.

Switzerland is the only country approaching Great Britain in freedom from restrictions. Voluntary enrichment is permitted subject to an upper limit (which there is not in Great Britain) and no claim may be made unless the food contains at least one-third RDI per serving. If it is claimed as a rich source the food must contain the full RDI. Authority is generally in favour of enrichment because of seasonal fluctuations in nutrient content and processing losses – a philosophy that appears to be unique to Switzerland.

Italy does not permit any foods to be enriched other than those designated dietetic foods which are sold through special stores; nothing is added to flour.

Enrichment in the United States is controlled and claims are subject to widespread regulations governing Food Labelling.

Such variations in regulations obviously present obstacles to international trade and harmonisation laws are under continuing discussion.

Developing Countries

There is a clear and urgent need for enrichment in many developing countries.

In India, for example, vitamin A deficiency is widespread. About 10–12 000 children go blind each year from xerophthalmia and one of the remedies is enrichment. Since tea is a universal drink, even by small children, this is used as a vehicle for enrichment. Small leaves, tea dust, are enriched by mixing with powdered retinol palmitate and only 15% is lost after 1 year storage. The stability is probably due to the antioxidants present in tea, including catechol, epicatechol, gallic acid, phenols and polyphenols.

Larger leaf tea is mixed with vitamin A acetate and palmitate. An emulsion in gum acacia or dextrin is mixed with 50% sucrose and sprayed on to the leaves. Loss is only 10% after 6 months' storage at 37°C.

The palmitate, but not the acetate, is completely stable when the tea is brewed.

The concentration is 37.5 μg vitamin A per g tea, and since 3 g is used per cup, this would provide 100 μg per cup. An adult drinking 3 cups per day would thus receive 300 μg towards the RDI of 750 μg, and a child drinking 1–2 cups would receive 110–220 μg.

In Guatemala vitamin A is being added to table sugar; some authorities have considered adding B vitamins to sugar on the principle that it makes a demand on the rest of the diet for the B vitamins needed for its metabolism.

An example of some of the principles and problems involved is provided by the enrichment of atta, the wheat flour used extensively in India for making chappatis, inaugurated in 1970. The Government accepted the difficulties in the way of changing food habits and used enrichment as the means of overcoming nutritional problems. Although most of the 20 million tons of wheat consumed per year is ground in small, hand-operated mills, three million tons pass through large mills and so can be enriched.

The following are added: edible grade groundnut flour (45–50% protein) 50 kg, retinol 9.2 g, riboflavin 1.38 g, niacin 7.6 g, thiamin 1.5 g, calcium diphosphate 800 g, iron as ferrous sulphate 96 g, calcium carbonate 800 g.

To prevent discolouration by reaction between the ferrous sulphate and phenolic substance in the groundnut flour the former is coated with starch. A pre-mix of all the nutrients in the groundnut flour is mixed with the atta at 5% level. Groundnut is tested for aflatoxin.

The cost in 1970 added 4% to the retail price and was subsidised for the early part of the programme. It was initiated in the flour mills of the major cities, to be spread, eventually to all mills.

Philosophy of enrichment

Some authorities accept enrichment only as a short-term policy pending improved food supplies, improved processing methods resulting in higher retention of nutrients, and nutritional education of the consumer.

Others regard it as a permanent policy and indeed, the Council for Foods and Nutrition of the American Medical Association has stated that efforts to improve the nutritional status of populations by the introduction of new foods and by attempts to change food habits often have not been effective.

Another aspect is the contention that foods should be enriched only with such nutrients as they already contain, although in inadequate amounts. In the United States the view has been expressed that to avoid undue artificiality of foods that are enriched, one should select only those that have suffered losses in processing and use only those in type or amount that are normally found in those foods. On these grounds permission has often been refused to U.S. manufacturers wishing to enrich proprietary foods.

Such views assume that unprocessed foods contain the nutrients required by man in the required proportions, as does the view that the nutritional profile of an unprocessed food must be preserved. It leads to the enrichment of fruit juices with vitamin C despite the fact that consumers of fruit juices will already be obtaining considerable amounts of this vitamin, while it is those who do not take such foods who may well be in short supply. It would therefore be logical to upset the nutritional profile and render some foods 'artificial' by adding the vitamin C to drinks like tea and coffee – such a policy, in fact, as has been accepted by the enrichment of tea with vitamin A in India and the enrichment of sugar.

Future developments

The Council on Foods and Nutrition of the American Medical Association classifies foods as conventional, formulated (mixtures of two or more foodstuffs or ingredients processed and blended together including breakfast cereals, convenience foods and snack foods) and fabricated (prepared principally from ingredients specifically designed to achieve a particular function not possible with common food ingredients).

The nutritional value of conventional foods can, they say, be improved by good processing practices. Restoration is acceptable when the product in question is nutritionally important, i.e. the nutrients originally present provided at least 5% RDI in a serving. 'Industry should strive to improve techniques rather than depend on restoration'.

When a formulated food has no easily identifiable counterpart among conventional foods and contributes 5% or more of the RDI of energy or any essential nutrient in one serving then nutrient additions should be related to the energy supplied, i.e. if it suppled 10% of the energy then it should supply the same percentage of the nutrients. If it already contains three-quarters of the nutrient then no adjustment is needed. A product designed primarily as a meal replacer should provide 25% to 50% of all nutrients listed in RDI tables except energy. Prepared breakfast cereals may be designed to provide up to 25% RDI per ounce, even if they are low energy foods for weight loss.

Fabricated foods may or may not closely resemble existing foods. If they do they should contain on an energy basis at least the variety and quantity (at least 75%) of nutrients contained in important amounts in the general class of foods to which the imitated food belongs.

A new food should provide one to one and a half times the representative RDI for important nutrients in relation to the energy intake. 'Selection of nutrients and the amounts used should be based upon the producer's suggested pattern of use of the food by consumers, the stability of the nutrients in the foods and good manufacturing practice'. (Council on Foods and Nutrition, American Medical Association).

Exceptions to these guide lines are made for dietetic foods.

For these purposes the U.S. Recommended Daily Allowances are used, which are derived on age and sex categories from the standard RDI figures.

The Report of the British Food Standard Committee on Novel Protein Foods in 1974 indicates possible developments for the future. It is clearly implied here that any new foods which are expected to replace traditional foods shall supply at least as much of the nutrient as the foods they replace. The obvious example is marketing of textured vegetable protein foods intended as alternatives to meat and the principle has already been applied in the case of margarine.

Since meat supplies a valuable portion of the thiamin, niacin, and vitamin B_{12}, and since the iron of meat is particularly well absorbed in contrast with the poor absorption from most other foods, such novel foods, it is suggested, should be enriched with these nutrients.

At the same time it is suggested that since the quality of the protein from soya, particularly after it has been spun or extruded, is below that of meat the finished product should have the sulphur amino acids brought up to the level found in meat.

Similar considerations will doubtless apply to all new products. Instant potato replaces a valuable source of vitamin C in many diets in the western countries and most manufacturers restore or even nutrify with vitamin C.

Changes in eating patterns may also call for enrichment as has been often suggested in the United States. For example, the break-up of the family eating pattern has often led to greater reliance on snack foods so that these need fortification if malnutrition is to be prevented.

For further literature see References 922–935.

References

MEAT AND MEAT PRODUCTS

1   Aitken, F. C. and Duncan, D. L. (1960). The vitamin content of carcase meat and other edible tissues and organs. *Nutr. Abst. Rev.* **30**, 743–779.

2   Baldwin, R. E., Korschgen, B. M., Russell, M. S. and Mabesa, L. (1976). Proximate analysis, free amino acid, vitamin and mineral content of microwave cooked meat. *J. Fd. Sci.* **41**, 762–765.

4   Bender, A. E. and Husaini. (1976). Nutritive value of proteins in a canned meat D. J. A. and Lawrie, R. A.). Butterworths, London.

4   Bender, A. E. and Husaini (1976). Nutritive value of proteins in a canned meat product. *J. Fd. Technol.* **11**, 499–504.

5   Bender, A. E. and Zia, M. (1976). Meat quality and protein quality. *J. Fd. Technol.* **11**, 495–498.

6   Beuk, J. F., Chornock, F. W. and Rice, E. E. (1948). The effect of severe heat treatment upon the amino acids of fresh and cured pork. *J. biol. Chem.* **175**, 291–297.

7   Beuk, J. F., Chornock, F. W. and Rice, E. E. (1949). The effect of heat on the availability of pork protein *in vivo* and *in vitro*. *J. biol. Chem.* **180**, 1243–1251.

8   Beuk, J. F., Fried, J. F. and Rice, E. E. (1950). Nutritive values of sausage and other table-ready meats as affected by processing. *Food Res.* **15**, 302–307.

9   Bowers, J. A. and Fryer, B.A. (1972). Thiamin and riboflavin in cooked and frozen reheated turkey. *J. Amer. Dietet. Assoc.* **60**, 399–401.

10   Boyle, M. A. and Funk, K. (1972). Thiamin in roast beef held by three methods. *J. Amer. Dietet. Assoc.* **60**, 398.

11   Burger, I. H. and Walters, C. L. (1973). The effect of processing on the nutritive value of flesh foods. *Proc. Nutr. Soc.* **32**, 1–8.

12   Carpenter, K. J., Ellinger, G. M. and Shrimpton, D. H. (1955). The evaluation of whaling by-products as feeding stuffs. *J. Sci. Fd. Agric.* **6**, 296–304.

13   Causey, K., Hausrath, M. E., Ramstad, P. E. and Fenton, F. (1950). Effect of thawing and cooking methods on the palatability and nutritive value of frozen ground meat. 1. Pork, 2. Beef, 3. Lamb. *Food Res.* **15**, 237–248, 249–255, 256–261.

14   Chang, I. C. L. (1952). The fatty acid content of meat and poultry before and after cooking. *J. Amer. Oil Chem. Soc.* **29**, 334, 378.

15   Clark, H. E. *et al.* (1955). The effect of braising and pressure saucepan cookery on the cooking losses, palatability and nutritive value of the proteins of round steaks. *Food Res.* **20**, 35–41.

16   Cole, L. N. (1962). The effect of storage at elevated temperature on some proteins of freeze-dried beef. *J. Fd. Sci.* **27**, 139.

17   Cook, B. B., Morgan, A. F.and Smith, M. B. (1949). Thiamine, riboflavin and niacin content of turkey tissue as effected by storage and cooking. *Food Res.* **14**, 449–458.

18   Cover, S., Dilsaver, E. M. and Hays, R. M. (1947). Retention of the B-vitamins in beef and lamb after stewing. 6. Similarities and differences among the four vitamins. *J. Amer. Dietet. Assoc.* **23**, 962–966.

19   Cover, S., Dilsaver, E. M., Hays, R. M. and Smith, W. H. (1949). Retention of B vitamins after large-scale cooking of meat. II Roasting by two methods. *J. Amer. Dietet. Assoc.* **25**, 949–954.

20   Cover, S., McClaren, B. A. and Pearson, P. B. (1944). Retention of B-vitamins in rare and well-done beef. *J. Nutr.* **27**, 363–375.

21   Cover, S. and Smith, W. H. (1948). Effect of thiamine retention of adding a carbohydrate vegetable to beef stew. *Food Res.* **13**, 475.

22   Cover, S. and Smith, W. H. (1956). Effect of moist and dry heat cooking on vitamin retention in meat from beef animals of different levels of fleshing. *Food Res.* **21**, 209–216.

23   Dunker, C. F., Berman, M., Snider, G. G. and Tubiash, H. S. (1953). Quality and nutritive properties of different types of commercially cured hams. III. Vitamin content, biological value of the protein and bacteriology. *Food. Technol.* **7**, 288–291.

24   Dvořák, Z. and Vognarová, I. (1965). Available lysine in meat and meat products. *J. Sci. Fd. Agric.* **16**, 305–312.

25   Dvořák, Z. and Vognarová, I. (1969). Nutritive value of the proteins of veal, beef and pork determined on the basis of available essential amino acids or hydroxyproline analysis. *J. Sci. Fd. Agric.* **20**, 146–150.

26   El-Gharbawi, M. I. and Dugan, L. R. (1965). Stability of nitrogenous compounds and lipids during storage of freeze-dried raw beef. *J. Fd. Sci.* **30**, 817–822.

27   Engler, P. P. and Bowers, J. A. (1975). Vitamin B$_6$ content of turkey cooked from frozen, partially frozen and thawed states. *J. Fd. Sci.* **40**, 615–617.

28   Engler, P. A. and Bowers, J. A. (1975). Vitamin B$_6$ in reheated, held and freshly cooked turkey breast. *J. Amer. Dietet. Assoc.* **67**, 42–44.

29   Erikson, S. E. and Boyden, R. E. (1947). Effect of different methods of cooking on the thiamine, riboflavin, and niacin content of pork: turkey. *Kentucky Agr. Expt. Sta. Bull.* **503**, 504.

30   Feaster, J. F., Jackson, J. M., Greenwood, D. A. and Kraybill, H. R. (1946). Vitamin retention in processed meat. Effect of storage. *Ind. Eng. Chem.* **38**, 87–89.

31   Feliciotti, E. and Esselen, W. B. (1957). Thermal destruction rates of thiamine in pureed meats and vegetables. *Food Technol.* **11**, 77–84.

32   Fishwick, M. J. and Zmarlicki, S. (1970). Freeze-dried turkey muscle. 1. Changes in nitrogenous compounds and lipids in dehydrated turkey muscle during storage. 2. Role of haem pigments as catalysts in the autoxidation of lipid constituents. *J. Sci. Fd. Agric.* **21**, 155–160, 160–163.

33   Greenwood, D. A., Beadle, B. W. and Kraybill, H. R. (1943). Stability of thiamine to heat. 2. Effect of meat-curing ingredients in aqueous solutions and in meat. *J. biol. Chem.* **149**, 349–354.

34   Greenwood, D. A., Kraybill, H. R., Feaster, J. F. and Jackson, J. M. (1944). Vitamin retention in processed meat: effect of thermal processing. *Ind. Eng. Chem.* **36**, 922–927.

35   Groninger, H. S., Tappel, A. L. and Knapp, F. W. (1956). Some chemical and organoleptic changes in gamma-irradiated meats. *Food Res.* **21**, 555–564.

36   Happich, M. L. *et al.* (1975). Composition and PER of partially dehydrated and defatted chopped beef and of partially defatted beef fatty tissue and combinations with selected proteins. *J. Fd. Sci.* **75**, 35–39.

37   Harries, J. M., Hubbard, A. W., Alder, F. E., Kay, M. and Williams, D. R. (1968). Studies on the composition of food. 3. The nutritive value of beef from intensively reared animals. *Brit. J. Nutr.* **22**, 21–31.

38   Herbert, L. S., Dillon, J. F., MacDonald, M. W. and Skurray, G. R. (1974). Batch-dry rendering: influence of processing conditions on meat meal quality. *J. Sci. Fd. Agric.* **25**, 1063–1070.

39   Hoagland, R., Hankins, O. G., Ellis, N. R. *et al.* (1947). Composition and nutritive value of hams as affected by method of curing. *Food Technol.* **1**, 540–552.

40   Hodson, A. Z. (1941). Effect of cooking on riboflavin in content of chicken meat. *Food Res.* **6**, 175–178.

41   Jackson, S. H., Crook, A., Malone, V. and Drake, T. G. H. (1945). The retention of thiamine, riboflavin and niacin in cooking pork and processing bacon. *J. Nutr.* **29**, 391–403.

43   Jarboe, J. K. and Mabrouk, A. F. (1974). Free amino acids, sugars and organic acids in aqueous beef extract. *J. Agric. Fd. Chem.* **22**, 787–791.

44   Karandaeva, V. P. (1964). Comparative nutritive values of meat dehydrated in a hot air drier and by freeze-drying. *Nutr. abstr. Rev.* **34**, 433.

45   Karmas, E., Thompson, J. E. and Peryman, D. B. (1962). Thiamin retention in freeze-dehydrated irradiated pork. *Food Techol.* **16** (3), 107.

46   Keller, J. D. and Kinsella, J. E. (1973). Phospholipid changes and lipid oxidation during cooking and frozen storage of raw ground beef. *J. Fd. Sci.* **38**, 1200–1204.

47   Kizlaitis, L., Deibel, C. and Siedler, A. J. (1964). Nutrient content of variety meats. II. Effects of cooking on vitamin A, ascorbic acid, iron, and proximate composition. *Food Technol.* **18**, 103–104.

48   Kondos, A. C. and McClymont, G. L. (1972). Nutritional evaluation of meat meals for poultry. *Aust. J. Agric. Res.* **23**, 913–922.

49   Kotschevar, L. H. (1955). B-vitamin retention in frozen meat. *J. Amer. Dietet. Assoc.* **31**, 589–596.

50   Larson, E. R. (1956). Vitamin losses in the drip from thawed frozen poultry. *J. Amer. Dietet. Assoc.* **32**, 716–718.

51   Lawrie, R. A. (1968). Chemical changes in meat due to processing. A review. *J. Sci. Food Agric.* **19**, 233–240.

52   Lee, F. A., Brooks, R. F., Pearson, A. M. *et al.* (1954). Effect of rate of freezing on pork quality. Appearance, palatability, and vitamin content. *J. Amer. Dietet. Assoc.* **30**, 351–354.

53   Lehrer, W. P., Weise, A. C., Harvey, W. R. and Moore, P. R. (1951). Effect of frozen storage and subsequent cooking on the thiamin, riboflavin and nicotinic acid content of pork chops. *Food Res.* **16**, 485–491.

54   Lehrer, W. P., Weise, A. C., Harvey, W. R. and Moore, P. R. (1952). The stability of thiamin, riboflavin and nicotinic acid of lamb chops during frozen storage and subsequent cooking. *Food Res.* **17**, 24–30.

55   Leverton, R. M. and Odell, G. V. (1958). The nutritive value of cooked meats. Oklahoma Agr. Exp. Sta. Misc. publ. MP. 45. Oklahoma State University, Stillwater.

56   Lushbough, C. H., Heller, B. S., Weir, E., Schweigert, B. S. (1962). Thiamine retention in meats after various heat treatments. *J. Amer. Diet. Ass.* **40**, 35–38.

57   Lushbough, C. H., Weichman, J. M. and Schweigert, B. S. (1959). The retention of vitamin B_6 in meat during cooking. *J. Nutr.* **67**, 451–459.

58   Mayfield, H. L. and Hedrick, M. T. (1949). The effect of canning, roasting and corning on the biological value of the proteins of western beef, finished on either grass or grain. *J. Nutr.* **37**, 487–494.

59   McBride, B. H., Guthneck, A. T., Hoffert, E. *et al.* (1951). Effect of frying bacon on the nutritive value of the protein. *J. Nutr.* **45**, 393–398.

60   Meyer, J. A., Briskey, E. J., Hoekstra, W. G. and Weckel, K. G. (1963).

Niacin, thiamine and riboflavin in fresh and cooked pale, soft, watery versus dark, firm, dry pork muscle. *Food Technol.* **17**, 485.
61   Meyer, B. H., Mysinger, M. A. and Buckley, R. (1963). The effect of three years of freezer storage on the thiamin, riboflavin and niacin content of ripened and unripened beef. *J. Agric. Fd. Chem.* **11**, 525–527.
62   Meyer, B. H., Mysinger, M. A. and Wodarski, L. A. (1969). Pantothenic acid and vitamin B_6 in beef. Retention after oven-roasting and oven-braising. *J. Amer. Dietet. Assoc.* **54**, 122–125.
63   Millares, R. and Fellers, C. R. (1949). Vitamin and amino acid content of processed chicken meat products. *Food Res.* **14**, 131–143.
64   Minoccheri, F. and Cantoni, C. (1971). B_1, B_2 and B_{12} vitamin content in Italian dry sausages and in seasoned hams. *Industrie Alimentari.* **10** (12), 76–79.
65   Minoccheri, F. and Cantoni, C. (1972). Vitamin levels in cooked sausages. *Industrie Alimentari.* **11**, 81. (*Food Manf.* **48**, 61, 1973.)
66   Morgan, A. F., Kidder, L. E., Hunner, M., Sharokh, B. K. and Chesbro, R. M. (1949). Thiamine, riboflavin and niacin content of chicken tissues, as affected by cooking and frozen storage. *Food Res.* **14**, 439–448.
67   Myers, S. J. and Harris, N. D. (1975). Effect of electronic cooking on fatty acid in meat. *J. Amer. Dietet. Assoc.* **67**, 232–234.
68   Newmark, H. L., Osadca, M. *et al.* (1974). Stability of ascorbate in bacon. *Food Technol.* **28**, 28–31.
69   Noble, I. (1964). Thiamine and riboflavin retention in broiled meat. Beef, lamb and pork. *J. Amer. Dietet. Assoc.* **45**, 447–450.
70   Noble, I. (1965). Thiamine and riboflavin retention in braised meat. *J. Amer. Dietet. Assoc.* **47**, 205.
71   Noble, I. (1970). Thiamin and riboflavin retention in cooked variety meats. *J. Amer. Dietet. Assoc.* **56**, 225.
72   Noble, I. and Gomez, L. (1958). Thiamine and riboflavin in roast lamb. *J. Amer. Dietet. Assoc.* **34**, 157–159.
73   Owen, J. E., Lawrie, R. A. and Hardy, B. (1975). Effect of dietary variation, with respect to energy and crude protein levels, on the oxidation activity exhibited by frozen porcine muscles. *J. Sci. Fd. Agric.* **26**, 31–41.
74   Pearson, A. M., Burnside, J. E., Edwards, H. M. *et al.* (1951). Vitamin losses in drip obtained upon defrosting frozen meat. *Food Res.* **16**, 85–87.
75   Pearson, A. M., Edwards, H. M., Burnside, J. E. *et al.* (1950). Vitamin losses in drip from frozen-defrosted beef. *J. Animal Sci.* **9**, 644–645.
76   Pellett, P. L. and Miller, D. S. (1963). The processing and preservation of meat in underdeveloped areas. *In* 'The better use of the world's fauna for food'. Institute of Biology, London.
77   Poling, C. E., Schultz, H. W. and Robinson, H. E. (1944). The retention of the nutritive quality of beef and pork muscle proteins during dehydration, canning, roasting and frying. *J. Nutr.* **27**, 23–34.
78   Pudelkewicz, C., Gordon, H., Whitworth, L. *et al.* (1963). Effects of processing and cooking on certain nutrients in fowl. Missouri Agric. Exp. Stat. Res. Bull. No. 819, p. 22.
79   Reedman, E. J. and Buckby, L. (1943). The vitamin B_1 content of canned pork. *Canad. J. Res.* **21**, 261–266.
80   Rice, E. E., Beuk, J. F. and Fried, J. F. (1947). Effect of commercial curing, smoking, storage and cooking operations upon vitamin content of pork hams. *Food Res.* **12**, 239–246.

81 Rice, E. E., Beuk, J. F. and Robinson, H. E. (1943). The stability of thiamin in dehydrated pork. *Science* **98**, 449.
82 Rice, E. E., Squires, E. M. and Fried, J. F. (1948). Effect of storage and microbial action on vitamin content of pork. *Food Res.* **13**, 195–202.
83 Robertson, J., Vipond, M. S., Tapsfield, D. and Greaves, J. P. (1966). Studies on the composition of food. 1. Some differences in the composition of broiler and free-range chickens. *Brit. J. Nutr.* **20**, 657–687.
84 Rognerud, G. (1972). Content of some nutrients in raw and prepared chicken. *Tidsskr. hermetikind.* **58**, 125. (In Norwegian.)
85 Rognerud, G. (1973). Contents of some nutrients in raw and prepared broilers. I. Thiamin, calcium and iron. *Nutr. Abstr. Rev.* **43**, No. 102.
86 Rowe, D. M., Mountrey, G. J. and Prudent, I. (1963). Effect of freeze-drying on thiamin, riboflavin and niacin content of chicken muscle. *Food Technol.* **17**, 1449–1450.
87 Sarrett, H. P. and Cheldelin, V. H. (1945). Thiamine, riboflavin and nicotinic acid retention in preparation of overseas hams and bacons. *J. Nutr.* **30**, 25–30.
88 Schroeder, L. J., Iacobellis, M. and Smith, A. H. (1961). Influence of heat on the digestibility of meat proteins. *J. Nutr.* **73**, 143–150.
89 Schweigert, B. S., Bennet, B. A., Marquette, M. *et al.* (1952). Thiamine, riboflavin and niacin content of processed meats. *Food Res.* **17**, 56–59.
90 Schweigert, B. S., McIntire, J. M. and Elvehjem, C. A. (1944). The retention of vitamins in pork hams during curing. *J. Nutr.* **27**, 419–424.
91 Schweigert, B. S. and Payne, B. J. (1956). A summary of the Nutrient Content of Meat. Bulletin No. 30, American Meat Inst. Foundation, Chicago.
92 Singh, S. P. and Essary, E. O. (1971). Vitamin content of broiler meat as affected by age, sex, thawing and cooking. *Poultry Sci.* **50**, 1150–1155.
93 Skurray, G. R. and Cumming, R. B. (1974a). Physical and chemical changes during batch dry rendering of meat meals. *J. Sci. Fd. Agric.* **25**, 521–527.
94 Skurray, G. R. and Cumming, R. B. (1974b). Prevention of browning during batch dry rendering. *J. Sci. Fd. Agric.* **25**, 529–533.
95 Skurray, G. R. and Herbert, L. S. (1974). Batch dry rendering: influence of raw materials and processing conditions on meat meal quality. *J. Sci. Fd. Agric.* **25**, 1071–1079.
96 Thomas, M. H. and Calloway, D. H. (1957). Nutritive value of irradiated turkey. *J. Amer. Dietet. Assoc.* **33**, 1030–1033.
96a Toepfer, E. W., Pritchett, C. A. and Hewston, E. M. (1955). Boneless beef; raw, cooked and stewed. *USDA Bull.* 1137.
97 Tucker, R. E., Hinman, W. F. and Halliday, E. G. (1946). The retention of thiamin and riboflavin in beef cuts during braising, frying and broiling. *J. Amer. Dietet. Assoc.* **22**, 877–881.
98 Vipond, M. S., Robertson, J. and Tapsfield, D. (1964). Some differences in composition of broiler and free-range chickens. *Proc. Nutr. Soc.* **23**, xxxviii.
99 Warner, W. D., Abell, P. N., Mone, P. E., Poling, C. E. and Rice, E. E. (1962). Nutritional value of fats in cooked meats. *J. Amer. Dietet. Assoc.* **40**, 422–426.
100 Webb, J. E., Brunson, C. C. and Yates, J. D. (1974). Effects of dietary fat and tocopherol on stability characteristics of frozen broiler parts. *J. Fd. Sci.* **39**, 133–136.
101 Westerman, B. D., Oliver, B. and Mackintosh, D. L. (1955). Influence of chilling rate and frozen storage on B-complex content of pork. *J. Agric. Fd. Chem.* **3**, 603–605.

102   Wheeler, P. and Morgan, A. F. (1958). The absorption by immature and adult rats of amino acids from raw and autoclaved fresh pork. *J. Nutr.* **64**, 137–150.
103   Whitmore, R. A., Pollard, A. E., Kraybill, H. R. and Elvehjem, C. A. (1946). Vitamin content of dehydrated meats. *Food Res.* **11**, 419–424.
104   Williams, J. C. (1936). Calcium in meat cooked with acid. *Food Res.* **1**, 537–549.
105   Younathan, M. T. and Watts, B. M. (1960). Oxidation of tissue lipids in cooked pork. *Food Res.* **25**, 538–543.

See also references 576, 578, 592, 597, 598, 603, 613, 625, 638, 642, 666, 663, 709.

FISH AND FISH PRODUCTS

106   Arnensen, G. (1969). Total and free amino acids in fishmeals, and vacuum-dried codfish organs, flesh, bones, skin and stomach contents. *J. Sci. Fd. Agric.* **20**, 218–220.
107   Bender, A. E. and Haizelden, S. (1957). Biological value of the proteins of a variety of fish meals. *Brit. J. Nutr.* **11**, 42–43.
108   Bisset, H. M. and Tarr, H. L. A. (1954). The effect of heating herring meals on their content in essential available amino acids. *Poult. Sci.* **33**, 250–254.
109   Blegen, E. and Wilsher, B. (1971). Nutrient contents in raw, deep frozen and prepared cod fillets. *Nutr. Abstr. Rev.* **41**, No. 2591.
110   Botta, J. R., Richards, J. F. and Tomlinson, N. (1973). Flesh pH, color, thaw drip, and mineral concentration of Pacific halibut (Hippoglossus stenolepis) and Chinook salmon (Oncorhynchus tshawytscha) frozen at sea. *J. Fisheries res. Board Canada.* **30**, 71–77.
111   Braekkan, O. R. and Boge, G. (1960). Biotin in Norwegian fish and fish products. *Tidsskr. hermetikind.* **46**, 467. (In Norwegian.)
112   Carpenter, K. J., Duckworth, J., Ellinger, G. M. and Shrimpton, D. H. (1952). The nutritional evaluation of protein concentrates obtained from the alkali digestion of herring. *J. Sci. Fd. Agric.* **3**, 278–288.
113   Carpenter, K. J., Lea, C. H. and Parr, L. J. (1963). Chemical and nutritional changes in stored herring meal. 4. Nutritional significance of oxidation of the oil. *Brit. J. Nutr.* **17**, 151–169.
114   Carpenter, K. J., Morgan, C. B., Lea, C. H. and Parr, L. J. (1962). Chemical and nutritional changes in stored herring meal. *Brit. J. Nutr.* **16**, 451–465.
115   Clandinin, D. R. (1949). The effects of methods of processing on the nutritive value of herring meals. *Poultry Sci.* **28**, 128–133.
116   Dubrow, D. and Hammerle, O. (1969). Holding raw fish (red hake) in IPA for FPC extraction. *Food Technol.* **23**, 254–256.
117   El-Lakany, S. and March, B. E. (1974). Chemical and nutritive changes in herring meal during storage at different temperatures with and without anti-oxidant treatment. *J. Sci. Fd. Agric.* **25**, 899–906.
118   Gurevič, G. P. (1966). Iodine in sea-fish differently processed. *Nutr. Abstr. Rev.* **36**, No. 2206.
119   Hallgren, B. (1970). Effect of processing on the nutritional value of fish protein concentrates. *In* 'Evaluation of Novel Protein Products'. Ed. Bender, A. E., Kihlberg, R., Löfqvist, B. and Munck, L. Pergamon Press, Oxford.
120   Kennedy, T. S. and Ley, F. T. (1971). Studies on the combined effects of

gamma radiation and cooking on the nutritive value of fish. *J. Sci. Fd. Agric.* **22**, 146–148.

121   Lea, C. H., Parr, L. J. and Carpenter, K. J. (1958). Chemical and nutritional changes in stored herring meal. *Brit. J. Nutr.* **12**, 297–312.

122   Lea, C. H., Parr, L. J. and Carpenter, K. J. (1960). Chemical and nutritional changes in stored herring meal. *Brit. J. Nutr.* **14**, 91–113.

123   Lovern, J. A. (1944). The effect of preservation process on the vitamin content of fish. *Proc. Nutr. Soc.* **2**, 100–104.

124   Mameesh, M. S., Boge, G., Myklestad, H. and Braekhan, O. R. (1966). Studies on the radiation preservation of fish. 1. The effect on certain vitamins in fresh fillet of cod and dogfish and in smoked fillets of cod and herring. *Nutr. Abstr. Rev.* **36**, No. 2282.

125   Meinke, W. W., Rahman, A. M. and Mattil, K. F. (1972). Some factors influencing the extraction of protein isolates from whole fish. *J. Fd. Sci.* **37**, 195.

126   Miller, D., Kifer, R. R. and Ambrose, M. E. (1970). Effects of storage on fish meal quality as evaluated by chemical indices and chick bioassay. *Poultry Sci.* **49**, 1005.

127   Miller, D. S. (1956). The nutritive value of fish proteins. *J. Sci. Fd. Agric.* **7**, 337–343.

128   Miller, E. L., Carpenter, K. J. and Milner, C. K. (1965). Availability of sulphur amino acids in protein foods. 3. Chemical and nutritional changes in heated cod muscle. *Brit. J. Nutr.* **19**, 547–564.

129   Miller, E. L., Hartley, A. W. and Thomas, D. C. (1965). Availability of sulphur amino acids in protein foods. 4. Effect of heat treatment upon the total amino acid content of cod muscle. *Brit. J. Nutr.* **19**, 565–573.

130   Moorjani, M. N., Nair, R. B. and Lahiry, N. L. (1968). Quality of fish protein concentrate prepared by direct extraction of fish with various solvents. *Food Technol.* **22**, 1557–1561.

131   Morrison, A. B. and Munro, I. C. (1965). Factors influencing the nutritional value of fish flour. IV. Reaction between 1,2-dichlorethane and protein. *Canad. J. Biochem.* **43**, 33–40.

132   Morrison, A. B. and Sabry, Z. I. (1963). Factors affecting the nutritional value of fish flour. *Can. J. Biochem. Physiol.* **41**, 649–655.

133   Morrison, A. B., Sabry, Z. I. and Middleton, E. J. (1962). Factors influencing the nutritional value of fish flour. I. Effects of extraction with chloroform or ethylene dichloride. *J. Nutr.* **77**, 97–104.

134   Munro, I. C. and Morrison, A. B. (1965). Effects of salting and smoking on protein quality of cod. *J. Fish Res. Bd. Canada.* **22**, 13–16.

135   Munro, I. C. and Morrison, A. B. (1967). Toxicity of 1,2-dichloroethane-extracted fish protein concentrate. *Canad. J. Biochem.* **45**, 1779–1781.

136   Myklestad, O., Bjørnstad, J. and Njaa, L. (1972). Effects of heat treatment on composition and nutritive value of herring meal. *Fiskerdinetoratets Skrifter Ser. Technol. Undersøk.* **5**, No. 10, 1–15. (In Norwegian.)

137   Quaglia, G. B., Audisio, P., Fabriani, G. and Fidanza, A. (1976). Effect of cooking on the fatty acid composition of the lipids of frozen fish on several species. 1. Composition in the total fatty acids. *Nutr. Abstr. Rev.* **46**, No. 53.

138   Rand, N. T., Collins, V. K., Varner, D. S. and Mosser, J. D. (1960). Biological evaluation of the factors affecting the protein quality of fish meals. *Poultry Sci.* **39**, 45–53.

139   Sen, D. P., Rao, T. S. S., Kadkol, S. B. *et al.* (1969). Fish protein concentrate

from Bombay duck fish (*Harpoden nehereus*); effect of processing variables in the nutritional and organoleptic qualities. *Food Technol.* **23**, 683–688.

140 Sinnhuber, R. O., Landers, M. K. and Yu, T. C. (1968). Radiation sterilisation of prefried cod and halibut patties. *Food Technol.* **22**, 1570–1572.

141 Srinivas, H., Vakil, U. K. and Sreenivasan, A. (1974). Nutritional and compositional changes in dehydro-irradiated shrimp. *J. Fd. Sci.* **39**, 807–811.

142 Tarr, H. L. A. (1969). Nutritional value of fish muscle and problems associated with its preservation. *Canad. Inst. Food Technol. J.* **2**, 42–45.

143 Tarr, H. L. A., Biely, J. and March, B. E. (1954). The nutritive value of herring meals. 1. The effect of heat. 2. Effect of heat on availability of essential amino acids. *Poultry Sci.* **33**, 242–250, 250–254.

144 Taarland, T., Mathiesen, E., Øosthus, Ø. and Braekkan, O. R. (1958). Nutritional values and vitamins of Norwegian fish and fish products. *Tidsskr. hermetikind.* **11**, 405–412. (In Norwegian.)

145 Tooley, P. J. (1972). Effect of deep fat frying on the availability of fish lysine. *Proc. Nutr. Soc.* **31**, 2A.

146 Tooley, P. J. and Lawrie, R. A. (1974). Effect of deep fat frying on availability of lysine in fish fillets. *J. Fd. Technol.* **9**, 247–253.

147 Torry Research Station (1970). Annual Report on the handling and preservation of fish and fish products, 1968. HMSO, London.

148 Varela, G., Pujol, A. and Moreiras-Varela, O. (1963). Biological value of protein in fresh and canned sardines. *Ann. Bromatol.* **15**, 117–125. (In Spanish.)

149 Yáñez, E., Ballester, D. and Donoso, G. (1970). Effects of drying temperature on the quality of fish protein. *J. Sci. Fd. Agric.* **21**, 426–428.

150 Yu, T. C., Landers, M. K. and Sinnhuber, R. O. (1969). Browning reaction in radiation-sterilised seafood products. *Food Technol.* **23**, 224–226.

See also references 621, 657, 763b, 832.

MILK

151 Aurand, L. W., Singleton, J. A. and Noble, B. W. (1966). Photo-oxidation reactions in milk. *J. Dairy Sci.* **49**, 138.

152 Bernhart, F. W., D'Amato, E. and Tomarelli, R. M. (1960). The vitamin B_6 activity of heat sterilised milk. *Arch. Biochem. Biophys.* **88**, 267–269.

153 Boatman, C. (1964). Effect of manufacturing conditions and storage on certain polyunsaturated fatty acids of dairy products. *J. Dairy Sci.* **47**, 194.

154 Brink, M. F., Baisley, M. and Speckman, E. W. (1969). Nutritional value of milk compared with filled and imitation milks. *Amer. J. Clin. Nutr.* **22**, 168–180.

155 Bujard, E., Handwerck, V. and Mauron, J. (1967). The differential determination of lysine in heated milk. I. *In vitro* methods. II. Comparison of the *in vitro* methods with biological evaluation. (Mottu, F. and Mauron, J.). *J. Sci. Food Agric.* **18**, 52–57, 57–62.

156 Bullock, D. M., Singh, S. and Pearson, A. M. (1968). Stability of vitamin C in enriched commercial evaporated milk. *J. Dairy Sci.* **50**, 920–923.

157 Burton, H., Ford, J. E., Perkin, A. G., Porter, J. W. G. *et al.* (1970). Comparison of milks processed by the direct and indirect methods of ultra-high temperature sterilisation. IV. The vitamin composition of milks sterilised by different processes. *J. Dairy Res.* **37**, 529–533.

158   Chapman, H. R., Ford, J. E., Kon, S. K., Thompson, S. Y. *et al.* (1957). Further studies on the effect of processing on some vitamins of the B complex in milk. *Dairy Res.* **24**, 191–197.
159   Conochie, J. and Wilkinson, R. A. (1958). The stability of vitamin A and carotene in fortified sweetened and condensed milk. *Aust. J. Dairy Tech.* **13**, 27–28.
160   Cook, B. B., Fraenkal-Conrat, J., Singer, B. and Morgan, A. F. (1951). The effect of heat treatment on the nutritive value of milk proteins. 3. The effect of heat on casein, lactalbumin and their lactose-induced derivatives with special reference to digestibility and the rate of release of lysine, methionine and tryptophan. *J. Nutr.* **44**, 217–235.
161   Cook, B. B., Morgan, A. F., Weast, F. O. and Parker, J. (1951). The effect of heat treatment on the nutritive value of milk proteins. 1. Evaporated and powdered milks. *J. Nutr.* **44**, 51–61, 63–81.
162   Davies, M. K., Gregory, M. E. and Henry, K. M. (1959). The effect of heat on the vitamin B_6 of milk. II. A comparison of biological and microbiological tests of evaporated milk. *J. Dairy Res.* **26**, 215–220.
163   Dimick, P. S. (1973). Effect of fluorescent light on the flavour and selected nutrients of homogenized milk held in conventional containers. *J. Milk Fd. Technol.* **36**, 383–387.
164   Dong, F. M. and Oace, S. M. (1975). Folate concentration and pattern and bovine milk. *J. Agric. Fd. Chem.* **23**, 534–538.
165   Dunkley, W. L., Franklin, J. D. and Pangborn, R. M. (1962). Effects of fluorescent light on flavour, ascorbic acid and riboflavin in milk. *Food Technol.* **16**, 112–118.
166   Eggum, B. O., Nielsen, H. E. and Rasmussen, F. L. (1970). Effect of storage on the protein quality of skim milk powder. *Ztschr. Tierphysiol. Tierernährung Futtermittelk.* **27**, 18–23.
167   Erbersdobler, H. and Dümmer, H. (1972). Analytical and physiological characteristics of amino acid damage after heat treatment. 3. Studies on an overheated milk powder. *Nutr. Abstr. Rev.* **42**, No. 8344.
168   Erbersdobler, H. and Zucker, H. (1966). Lysine and available lysine in dried skim milk. *Milchwissenschaft* **21**, 564–568. (In German.)
169   Fairbanks, B. W. and Mitchell, H. H. (1935). The nutritive value of skim milk powders, with special reference to the sensitivity of milk proteins to heat. *J. Agric. Res.* **51**, 1107–1121.
170   Ford, J. E. (1969). Effects of ultra-high-temperature (UHT) processing and of subsequent storage on the vitamin content of milk. *J. Dairy Res.* **36**, 447.
171   Ford, J. E., Porter, J. W. G., Scott, K. J. *et al.* (1974). Comparison of dried milk preparations for babies on sale in 7 European countries. II. Folic acid, vitamin B_6, thiamin, riboflavin and vitamin E. *Arch. Dis. Childh.* **49**, 874–877.
172   Ford, J. E., Porter, J. W. G., Thompson, S. Y. *et al.* (1968). Effects of UHT-processing and subsequent storage on the vitamin content of milk. *Proc. Nutr. Soc.* **27**, 60A–61A.
173   Ford, J. E. and Scott, K. J. (1968). The folic acid activity of some milk foods for babies. *J. Dairy Res.* **35**, 85–90.
174   Graham, D. M. (1974). Alteration of nutritive value resulting from processing and fortification of milk products. *J. Dairy Sci.* **57**, 738–745.
175   Gregory, M. E. (1975). Water-soluble vitamins in milk and milk products. *J. Dairy Res.* **42**, 197–216.

176   Gregory, M. E. and Burton, H. (1965). The effect of ultra-high-temperature heat treatment on the content of thiamine, vitamin B_6 and vitamin B_{12} of milk. *J. Dairy Res.* **32**, 13–17.

177   Gregory, M. E., Hansen, A. P. and Aurand, L. W. 1972). Controlling light-activated flavour in milk. *Amer. Dairy Rev.* **34** (4): 10, 11, 47–50.

178   Gregory, M. E., Henry, K. M., Kon, S. K. *et al.* (1961). The effect of hydrogen peroxide on the nutritive value of milk. *J. Dairy Sci.* **28**, 177–182.

179   Gregory, M. E., Henry, K. M. and Kon, S. K. (1964). Nutritional properties of freshly prepared and stored evaporated milks manufactured by a normal commerical procedure or by reduced thermal process in the presence of nisin. *J. Dairy Res.* **31**, 113.

179a Grudskaja, O. (1965). Effect of technological treatment on the ascorbic acid content of milk. *Nutr. Abstr. Rev.* **35**, 76.

180   Hedrick, T. I. (1969). New and special dairy products and processes. *Dairy Industr.* **34**, 420–425.

181   Hedrick, T. I. and Glass, L. (1975). Chemical changes in milk during exposure to fluorescent light. *J. Milk Food Technol.* **38**, 129–131.

182   Henry, K. M., Houston, J., Kon, S. K. and Thompson, S. Y. (1944). The effects of commercial processing and storage on some nutritive properties of milk. Comparison of full-cream sweetened condensed milk and of evaporated milk with original raw milk. *J. Dairy Res.* **13**, 329–339.

183   Henry, K. M. and Kon, S. K. (1947-48). Deterioration on storage of dried skim milk. IV. Changes in the biological value of the proteins. *J. Dairy Res.* **15**, 341.

184   Henry, K. M., Kon, S. K., Lea, C. H. and White, J. C. D. (1948). Deterioration on storage of dried skim milk. *J. Dairy Res.* **15**, 292–363.

185   Henry, K. M., Kon, S. K. and Watson, M. B. (1937). The effect of commercial pasteurisation on the biological value and digestibility of the proteins (nitrogen) of milk. 'Milk and Nutrition', Part 1. *Nat. Inst. for Dairying Report*, Pub. No. 37.

186   Hetrick, J. H. (1969). Imitation dairy products past, present and future. *J. Amer. Oil Chem. Soc.* **46**, 58A, 60A, 62A.

187   Hodson, A. Z. and Krueger, G. M. (1947). Changes in the essential amino acid content of the proteins of dry skim milk on prolonged storage. *Arch. Biochem.* **12**, 51–55.

188   Holland, R. F. (1969). Flavour, nutritional values of filled and imitation milks. *Amer. Dairy Rev.* **31**, 60–69.

189   Holmes, A. D. (1949). Decrease of reduced ascorbic acid in goat's milk during storage. *Food Res.* **16**, 468–471.

190   Holmes, A. D. and Jones, C. P. (1964). Effect of sunshine upon the ascorbic acid and riboflavin content of milk. *J. Nutr.* **29**, 201–209.

191   Holmes, A. D., Kuzmeski, J. W. and Canavan, F. T. (1946). Stability of vitamins in stored ice cream. *J. Amer. Dietet. Assoc.* **22**, 670–672.

192   Kon, S. K. (1938). The effect of commercial sterilisation on the nutritive value of milk. 7. Conclusions. *J. Dairy Res.* **9**, 185–207.

193   Kon, S. K. (1944). The chemical composition and nutritive value of milk and milk products. *Proc. Nutr. Soc.* **2**, 149–157.

194   Kon, S. K. (1960). Nutritional effects on milk of chemical additives and processing. 5th Int. Congr. on Nutr., Washington, panel VI. *Fed. Proc.* **20**, Part III, 209.

195   Kon, S. K. (1961). Nutritional effects on milk of chemical additives and processing. *Fed. Proc.* **20**, Suppl. 7, Part III, 209–216.

196 Lyster, F. L. J. (1965). Composition of milk deposits in an ultra-high temperature plant. *J. Dairy Res.* **32**, 203–208.

197 Mauron, J., Mottu, F., Bujard, E. and Egli, R. H. (1955). The availability of lysine, methionine and tryptophan in condensed milk and milk powder *in vitro* digestion studies. *Arch. Biochem. Biophys.* **59**, 433–451.

198 Moore, J. H. and Williams, D. L. (1965). A note on the effect of a commercial drying process on the long chain fatty acids of milk. *J. Dairy Res.* **32**, 19-20.

199 Pasricha, S. (1969). Effect of curdling on the thiamin, riboflavin and nicotinic acid content of milk. *J. Nutr. Dietet.* (*India*) **6**, 196–199.

200 Patton, S. (1954). The mechanism of sunlight-flavor formation in milk with special reference to methionine and riboflavin. *J. Dairy Sci.* **37**, 446.

201 Pol, G. and de Groot, E. H. (1960). Effect of processing on the nutritive value of milk. *Nederlands Melk Zuiveltijdschr.* **14**, 158–175. (In Dutch.)

202 Porter, J. W. G. and Thompson, S. Y. (1969). Effect of heat treatment on the nutritive quality of liquid milk, with particular reference to UHT (ultra heat treatment) processes. *Dtsch. Ges. Chem. Apparat. Monogr.* **63**, 233–241.

202a Porter, J. W. G. and Thompson, S. Y. (1976). Effects of processing on the nutritive value of milk. *Proc. 4th Internat. Cong. Fd. Sci. Technol.* Madrid. Vol. 1.

203 Posati, L. P., Holsinger, V. H., DeVilbiss, E. D. and Pallansch, M. J. (1974). Effect of instantizing on amino acid content of non-fat dry milk. *J. Dairy Sci.* **57**, 258–260.

204 Reiser, R. (1969). Nutritional inferiority of filled versus natural milk with special reference to fatty constituents. *J. Dairy Sci.* **52**, 1127–1129.

205 Rolls, B. A. and Porter, J. W. G. (1973). Some effects of processing and storage on the nutritive value of milk and milk products. *Proc. Nutr. Soc.* **32**, 9–15.

206 Sattar, A. and de Man, J. M. (1973). Effect of packaging material on light-induced quality deterioration of milk. *Canad. Inst. Food Sci. and Tech. J.* **6** (3), 170.

207 Schiller, K. (1956). Changes in skimmed milk powder during storage. *Ztschr. Tiernähr. Futtermittelk.* **11**, 264–267. (In German.)

208 Schroeder, L. J., Iacobellis, M. and Smith, A. H. (1953). Heat processing and the nutritive value of milk and milk products. *J. Nutr.* **49**, 549–561.

209 Singh, R. P., Heldman, D. R. and Kirk, J. R. (1975). Kinetic analysis of light-induced riboflavin loss in whole milk. *J. Fd. Sci.* **40** (1), 164–167.

210 Stull, J. W. (1953). The effect of light on activated flavour development and on the constituents of milk and its products. A review. *J. Dairy Sci.* **36**, 1153–1164.

211 Sweetsur, A. W. M. and White, J. C. D. (1976). Studies on the heat stability of milk protein. II. Effect of exposing milk to light. *J. Dairy Res.* **42**, 57–71.

212 Thompson, S. Y. (1968). Reviews of the progress of dairy science. Section D. Nutritive value of milk and milk products. Fat-soluble vitamins in milk and milk products. *J. Dairy Res.* **35**, 149.

213 Thompson, J. N. and Erdoby, P. (1974). Destruction by light of vitamin A added to milk. *J. Canad. Inst. Fd. Technol.* **7**, 157–158.

214 Van Den Beuel, A., Jamnskens, P. and Mol, J. (1972). Availability of lysine in skim milk powders processed under various conditions. *Neth. Milk Dairy J.* **26**, 19.

215 Whitnah, C. H. (1943). Nutritive value of milk proteins. *Food Res.* **8**, 89–94.

216 Withycombe, D. A. and Lindsay, R. C. (1969). Evidence of losses of free fatty acids in heated milk. *J. Dairy Sci.* **52**, 1100–1104.

217 Woodring, M. J. and Storvick, C. A. (1960). Vitamin B_6 in milk; Review of literature. *J. Assoc. Off. agric. Chem.* **43**, 63–80.

CEREALS

218 Aykroyd, W. R., Krishnan, B. G., Passmore, R. and Sundararajan, A. R. (1940). *Indian med. Res. Mem.* No. 32.

219 Barber, S. (1972). Milled rice and changes during aging. *In* 'Rice Chemistry and Technology'. Ed. D. F. Houston, Amer. Assoc. Cereal Chem., St. Paul, Minn.

220 Bayfield, E. G. and O'Donnell, W. W. (1945). Observations on thiamin content of stored wheat. *Food Res.* **10**, 485–488.

221 Blamberg, D. C. (1970). Protein quality of dry breakfast cereals. *Nutr. Report Intl.* **2**, 291–296.

222 Blessin, C. W., Cavins, J. F. and Inglett, G. E. (1971). Lysine-infused popcorn. *Cereal Chem.* **48**, 373–377.

223 Bressani, R., Castillo, S. V. and Guzman, M. A. (1962). The nutritional evaluation of processed whole corn flours. *J. Agric. Fd. Chem.* **10**, 308–312.

224 Bressani, R., Paz y Paz, R. and Scrimshaw, N. S. (1958). Chemical changes in corn during preparation of tortillas. *J. Agric. Fd. Chem.* **6**, 770–774.

225 Briant, A. M. and Klosterman, A. M. (1950). Influence of ingredients on thiamine and riboflavin retention and quality of plain muffins. *Trans. Am. Assoc. Cereal Chem.* **8**, 69.

226 Bunting, W. R. (1965). The stability of pyridoxine added to cereals. *Cereal Chem.* **42**, 569–572.

227 Burt, A. W. A. (1973). The effect of processing on the nutritive value of cereal in animal feeds. *Proc. Nutr. Soc.* **32**, 31–39.

228 Cailleau, R., Kidder, L. E. and Morgan, A. F. (1945). The thiamine content of raw and parboiled rices. *Cereal Chem.* **22**, 50–60.

229 Calhoun, W. K., Hepburn, F. N., Bradley, W. B. (1960). The availability of lysine in wheat flour, bread and gluten. *J. Nutr.* **70**, 337–347.

230 Carnovale, E., Fabriani, G., Fratoni, A. and Quaglia, G. B. (1969). Effect of processing and cooking on amino acid content of food pastes. *Quad. Nutrizione* **29**, 41–52.

231 Carpenter, K. J. and March, B. E. (1961). The availability of lysine in groundnut biscuits used in the treatment of kwashiorkor. *J. Nutr.* **15**, 403–410.

232 Chamberlain, N., Collins, T. H., Elton, G. A. H. *et al.* (1966). Studies on the composition of food. 2. Comparison of the nutrient content of bread made conventionally and by the Chorleywood bread process. *Brit. J. Nutr.* **20**, 747–755.

233 Chappel, C. I. and MacQueen, K. F. (1970). Effect of gamma radiation on vitamin content of enriched flour. *Food Irradiation* **10**, 8–10.

234 Chaudri, A. B. and Muller, H. G. (1974). The destruction of thiamin during chapati baking. *J. Fd. Technol.* **9**, 123–124.

235 Chow, C. K. and Draper, H. H. (1969). Effect of artificial drying on tocopherol and fatty acids in corn. *J. Agric. Fd. Chem.* **17**, 1316–1317.

236 Clarke, H. E., Howe, J. M., Mertz, E. T. and Reitz, L. L. (1959). Lysine in baking powder biscuits. *J. Amer. Dietet. Assoc.* **35**, 469–471.

237 Clegg, K. M. (1960). The availability of lysine in groundnut biscuits used in the treatment of kwashiorkor. *Brit. J. Nutr.* **14**, 325–329.

238 Clegg, K. M. (1963). Bound nicotinic acid in dietary wheaten products. *Brit. J. Nutr.* **17**, 325–329.

239 Coppock, J. B. M., Carpenter, B. R. and Knight, R. A. (1957). Cereal product fortification; the B vitamins with special reference to thiamine losses in baked products. *J. Sci. Fd. Agric.* **7**, 457–464.

240 Cort, W. M., Borenstein, B., Harley, J. H., Osadca, M. and Scheiner, J. (1976). Nutrient stability of fortified cereal products. *Food Technol.* **30**, 52–62.

241 Cuendet, L. S., Larson, E., Norris, C. G. and Geddes, W. F. (1954). The influence of moisture content and other factors on the stability of wheat flour at 37.8°C. *Cereal Chem.* **31**, 362–389.

242 Daniels, N. W. R., Russel Eggitt, P. W. and Coppock, J. B. M. (1960). Studies on the lipids of flour. 1. Effect of chlorine dioxide treatment on the essential fatty acids. *J. Sci. Fd. Agric.* **11**, 658–664.

243 Dawson, E. R. and Martin, G. W. (1942). Vitamin B_1. Estimation in wholemeal and brown bread and stability of different forms of vitamin B_1 during bread making. *J. Soc. Ind. Chem.* **61**, 13–18.

244 Downs, D. E. and Meckel, R. B. (1943). Thiamin losses in toasting bread. *Cereal Chem.* **20**, 352–355.

245 Ericson, L. E., Larsson, S. and Lid, G. (1961). The loss of added lysine and threonine during the baking of wheat bread. *Acta. Physiol. Scand.* **53**, 85.

246 Ferrel, R. E., Shepherd, A. D. and Guadagni, D. G. (1970). Storage stability of lysine in lysine-fortified wheat. *Cereal Chem.* **47**, 33–37.

247 Frazer, A. C. and Lines, J. G. (1967). Studies on changes in flour tocopherols following ageing and treatment of the flour with chlorine dioxide. *J. Sci. Fd. Agric.* **18**, 203–207.

248 Golberg, L. and Thorp, J. M. (1946). Loss of thiamin during baking of bread. *Nature* **158**, 22–23.

249 Gorbach. G. and Regula, E. (1964). The loss of essential amino acids in the baking process. *Fette: Seifen: Anstrichmittel* **66**, 920–925. (In German.)

250 Gotthold, N. L. M. and Kennedy, B. M. (1964). Biological evaluation of protein in steamed and baked breads and in bread ingredients. *J. Fd. Sci.* **29**, 227–232.

251 Hackler, L. R. (1972). Nutritional evaluation of protein quality in breakfast foods. *Cereal Chem.* **49**, 677–683.

252 Hepburn, F. N., Calhoun, W. K. and Bradley, W. B. (1966). The biological availability of essential amino acids in wheat, flour, bread and gluten. *Cereal Chem.* **43**, 271–283.

253 Herting, D. C. and Drury, E. E. (1969). Alpha-tocopherol content of cereal grains and processed cereals. *J. Agric. Fd. Chem.* **17**, 785–790.

254 Houston, D. F. and Kohler, G. O. (1970). Nutritional properties of rice. Food & Nutrition Board, Nat. Res. Council – Nat. Acad. Sci., Washington, DC.

255 Hutchinson, J. B., Moran, T. and Pace, J. (1964). The effect of a steam treatment on the feeding value of wheat. *J. Sci. Fd. Agric.* **15**, 413–417.

256 Jansen, G. R., Ehle, S. R. and Hause, N. L. (1964a). Studies of the nutritive loss of supplemented lysine in baking. 1. Loss in a standard white bread containing 4% nonfat dry milk. *Food. Technol.* **18**, 109–113.

257 Jansen, G. R., Ehle, S. R. and Hause, N. L. (1964b). Studies on the nutritive loss of supplemental lysine in baking. II. Loss in water bread and in breads supplemented with moderate amounts of nonfat dry milk. *Food Technol.* **18**, 114–117.

258 Jansen, G. R., Ehle, S. R. and Hause, N. L. (1964c). Studies on the nutritive loss of supplemented lysine in baking. *Food Technol.* **18**, 367–372.

259 Keagy, P. M., Stokstad, E. L. R. and Fellers, D. (1975). Folacin stability during bread processing and family flour storage. *Cereal Chem.* **52**, 348–356.

260 Kik, M. C. (1945). Effect of milling, processing, washing, cooking and storage on thiamine, riboflavin and niacin in rice. *Arkansas Agric. Expt. Sta. Bull.* 458

261 Kik, M. C. (1955). Influence of processing on the nutritive value of milled rice. *J. Agric. Fd. Chem.* **3**, 600–603.

262 Kik, M. C. and Williams, R. R. (1945). The nutritional improvement of white rice. *Bull. Nat. Res. Counc.* No. 112 (Washington, USA).

263 Knight, R. A., Christie, A. A., Orton, C. R. and Robertson, J. (1973). Studies on the composition of food. 4. Comparison of the nutrient content of retail white bread made conventionally and by the Chorleywood Bread Process. *Brit. J. Nutr.* **30**, 181–188.

264 Kondo, M. and Okamura, T. (1933 & 1934). Storage of rice. *Ber. Ohara Inst. Landwirtsch. Forsch.* **5**, 395–420: **6**, 149–174; 175–185.

265 Kuether, C. A. and Meyers, V. C. (1948). The nutritive value of cereal proteins in human subjects. *J. Nutr.* **35**, 651–667.

265a Laporte, T. and Trémolières, J. (1962). *C. R. Soc. Biol.* **156**, 1261.

266 Lincoln, H., Hove, E. L. and Harrel, C. G. (1944). The loss of thiamine on cooking breakfast cereals. *Cereal Chem.* **21**, 274–279.

267 Linko, Y. and Johnson, J. A. (1963). Non-enzymatic bread browning and flavour changes in amino acids and formation of carbonyl compounds during baking. *J. Agric. Fd. Chem.* **11**, 150–152.

268 Loy, H. W., Haggerty, J. F. and Combs, E. L. (1951). Light destruction of riboflavin in bakery products. *Food Res.* **16**, 360–364.

269 Maleki, M. and Djazayeri, A. (1968). Effect of baking and amino acid supplementation on the protein quality of Arabic bread. *J. Sci. Fd. Agric.* **19**, 449–451.

270 Mauron, J., Mottu, F. and Egli, R. H. (1960). Nutritional problems underlying protein malnutrition in developing countries. 1. Loss of amino acids in preparation of biscuits rich in protein. *Ann. Nutr. Alimentation* **14**, 135–150.

271 Metta, V. C. and Johnson, B. C. (1959). Biological value of gamma irradiated corn protein and wheat gluten. *J. Agric. Fd. Chem.* **7**, 131–133.

271a Miladi, S., Hegsted, D. M., Saunders, R. M. and Kohler, G. O. (1972). The relative nutritive value, amino acid content and digestibility of the protein of wheat mill fractions. *Cereal Chem.* **49**, 119–127.

272 Milner, C. K. and Carpenter, K. J. (1969). Effect of wet heat-processing on the nutritive value of whole-wheat protein. *Cereal Chem.* **46**, 425–434.

273 Mitchell, H. H. and Beadles, J. R. (1949). The effect of storage on the nutritional qualities of the proteins of wheat, corn and soybean. *J. Nutr.* **39**, 463–484.

274 Moran, T. (1959). Nutritional significance of recent work on wheat flour and bread. *Nutr. Abstr. Rev.* **29**, 1–16.

275 Mossman, A. P., Rockwell, W. C. and Fellers, D. A. (1973). Hot air toasting and rolling whole wheat. Effect on organoleptic, physical and nutritional quality. *J. Fd. Sci.* **38**, 879–884.

276 Murlin, J. R., Nasset, E. C. and Marsh, B. E. (1938). The egg–replacement value of the proteins of cereal breakfast foods, with a consideration of heat injury. *J. Nutr.* **16**, 249–269.

277 Ofosu, A. (1971). Changes in the levels of niacin and lysine during the traditional preparation of kenkey from maize grain. *Ghana J. Agric. Sci.* **4**, 153–158.

278 Ostwald, R. (1963). Fat content and fatty acids in some commercial mixes for baked products. *J. Amer. Dietet. Assoc.* **42**, 32–36.
279 Pace, J. K. and Whitacre, J. (1953). Factors affecting retention of B vitamins in corn bread made with enriched meal. III. Retention of thiamine in corn muffins made with commercial mixes and in corn bread made with self rising meals. *Food Res.* **18**, 231–238; 239–244; 245–249.
280 Padua, A. B. and Juliano, B. O. (1974). Effect of parboiling on thiamin, protein and fat of rice. *J. Sci. Fd. Agric.* **25**, 697–701.
281 Parker, H. K. (1960). Continuous breadmaking processes. *In* 'Bakery Technology and Engineering'. Ed. Matz, S.A. Avi Publishing Co., Westport, Conn.
282 Prabhavathi, C., Osha, M. S. and Bains, G. S. (1973). Effect of baking on the protein quality of high protein biscuits. *Ind. J. Nutr. Dietet.* **10**, 91–95.
283 Pujol, A. and Gonzalez, F. (1968). Disinfestation of cereals by ^{137}Cs gamma-radiation and biological value of the proteins of irradiated wheat flour. *Ann. Bromatol.* **20**, 149–182. (In Spanish.)
284 Rosenberg, H. R. and Rohdenburg, E. L. (1951). The fortification of bread with lysine. 1. The loss of lysine during baking. *J. Nutr.* **45**, 593–598.
285 Roy, J. K. and Rao, R. K. (1963). Alkalinity of cooking water and stability of rice. *Indian J. Med. Res.* **51**, 533.
286 Sabry, Z. I. and Tannous, R. I. (1961). Effect of parboiling on the thiamine, riboflavin and niacin contents of wheat. *Cereal Chem.* **38**, 536–539.
287 Schultz, A. S., Atkin, L. and Frey, C. N. (1942). The stability of vitamin B_1 in the manufacture of bread. *Cereal Chem.* **19**, 532–538.
288 Shyamala, G. and Kennedy, B. M. (1962). Protein value of chapatis and puris. *J. Amer. Dietet. Assoc.* **41**, 115–118.
289 Shyamala, G. and Lyman, R. L. (1964). The isolation and purification of a trypsin inhibitor from whole wheat flour. *Can. J. Biochem. Physiol.* **42**, 1825.
290 Slover, H. T. and Lehmann, J. (1972). Effect of fumigation on wheat in storage. 4. Tocopherols. *Cereal Chem.* **49**, 412–415.
291 Sowbhagya, C. M. and Bhattacharya, K. R. (1976). Lipid autoxidation in rice. *J. Fd. Sci.* **41**, 1018–1023.
292 Squibb, R. L., Braham, J. E., Arroyave, G., Scrimshaw, N. S. (1959). A comparison of the effects of raw corn and tortillas (lime-treated corn) with niacin, tryptophan or beans on the growth and muscle niacin of rats. *J. Nutr.* **67**, 351–361.
293 Stephens, L. C. and Chastain, M. F. (1959). Light destruction of riboflavin in partially baked rolls. *Food Technol.* **13**, 527–528.
294 Stewart, R. A., Hensley, G. W. and Peters, F. N. (1943). The nutritive value of protein. 1. The effect of processing on oat protein. *J. Nutr.* **26**, 519–526.
295 Sure, B. (1951). Nutritional value of proteins in various cereal breakfast foods. *Food Res.* **16**, 161–165.
296 Swaminathan, M. (1942). The effect of washing and cooking on the vitamin B_1 content of raw and parboiled rice. *Ind. J. Med. Res.* **30**, 409.
297 Tara, K. A. and Bains, G. S. (1971). Effects of cooking rice on the stability of lysine and threonine in a model system. *Ind. J. Nutr. Dietet.* **8**, 186–188.
298 Thewlis, B. H. (1971). Fate of ascorbic acid in the Chorleywood bread process. *J. Sci. Fd. Agric.* **22**, 16–19.
299 Tichenor, D. A., Martin, D. C. and Wells, C. E. (1965). Carotenoid content of frozen and irradiated sweet corn. *Food Technol.* **19**, 406–409.

300 Toepfer, E. W. *et al.* (1972). Nutrient composition of selected wheats and wheat products. XI. Summary. *Cereal Chem.* **49**, 173–186.
301 Valtadoros, A. (1976). Protein enrichment of wheat and its products; nutritional and technological aspects. *Proc. 4th Internat. Cong. Fd. Sci. Technol.* Madrid. Vol. 1.
302 Vojnovich, C. and Pfeifer, V. F. (1970). Stability of ascorbic acid in blends with wheat flour, CSM and infant cereals. *Cereal Sci. Today* **15**, 317–322.
303 Wall, J. S., James, C. and Cavins, J. F. (1971). Nutritive value of protein in hominy feed fractions. *Cereal Chem.* **48**, 456.
304 Washüttl, J. (1971). Free and bound tryptophan in wheat after gamma-irradiation. *Ernährungs-Umschau.* **18**, 98–100.
305 Womack, M., Vaughan, D. A. and Miller, L. R. (1974). Nutritive value of breakfast cereal-milk combination. *J. Fd. Sci.* **39**, 371–373.
306 Zaehringer, M. V. and Personius, C. J. (1949). Thiamine retention in bread and rolls baked to different degrees of browness. *Cereal Chem.* **26**, 384–392.
307 Zeleny, L. (1960). Cereal grains, P. 368. *In* 'Nutritional Evaluation of Food Processing'. Ed. R. S. Harris and H. von Loesecke. John Wiley and Sons, London.

See also references 555, 593, 602, 622, 626, 650, 652, 661, 703, 706, 731, 743, 812, 885, 922, 935.

FRUIT AND FRUIT PRODUCTS AND VEGETABLES

308 Abrams, C. I. (1975). The ascorbic acid content of quick frozen Brussels sprouts. *J. Fd. Technol.* **10**, 203–213.
309 Adam, W. B. (1941). Rep. Fruit Veg. Preserv. Res. Stn. 14.
310 Allen, R. J. L., Barker, J. and Mapson, L. W. (1943). The drying of vegetables. 1. Cabbage. *J. Soc. Chem. Ind.* **62**, 145–160.
311 Ang, C. Y. W. and Livingstone, G. E. (1974). Nutritive losses in the home storage and preparation of raw fruits and vegetables. *In* 'Nutritional qualities of fresh fruits and vegetables'. Ed. White, P. L. and Silvey, N. P. **51**. Futura Publ. Co. N.Y. U.S.A.
312 Bauernfeind, J. C., Osadca, M. and Bunnell, R. H. (1962). β-Carotene, colour and nutrient for juices and beverages. *Food Technol.* **16**, No. 8, 101–108.
313 Bender, A. E. (1958). The stability of vitamin C in a commercial fruit squash. *J. Sci. Fd. Agric.* **11**, 754–760.
313a Bender, A. E., Getreuer, A. and Harris, M. (1977). Feeding of school children in a London borough. *Brit. Med. J.* **1**, 757–759.
314 Berry, R. E., Bissett, O. W. and Veldhuis, M. K. (1971). Vitamin C retention in orange juice as related to container type. *Citrus Industr.* **52**, 12–13.
315 Birch, G. G., Bointon, B. M., Rolfe, E. J. and Selman, J. D. (1974). Quality changes involving vitamin C in fruit and vegetable processing. *In* 'Vitamin C'. Ed. Birch, G. G. and Parker, K. J. Applied Science Publishers Ltd., London.
316 Bissett, O. W. and Berry, R. E. (1975). Ascorbic acid retention in orange juice as related to container type. *J. Fd. Sci.* **40**, 178–180.
317 Booth, V. H. and Bradford, M. P. (1963). Effects of cooking on alpha-tocopherol in vegetables. *Internat. Ztschr. Vitaminforsch.* **33**, 276–278.
318 Burger, M., Hein, L. W., Teply, L. J. *et al.* (1956). Vitamin, mineral and

proximate composition of frozen fruits, juices and vegetables. *J. Agric. Fd. Chem.* **4**, 418–425.

319 Cain, R. F. (1967). Water soluble vitamins: changes during processing and storage of fruits and vegetables. *Food Technol.* **21**, 998–1007.

320 Chan, H. T., Kwo, M. T., Cavaletto, C. G., Nakayama, T. O. M. and Brekke, J. E. (1975). Papaya purée and concentrate: change in ascorbic acid, carotenoids and sensory quality during processing. *J. Fd. Sci.* **40**, 701–703.

321 Chick, H. and Dalyell, E. J. (1920). The influence of overcooking vegetables in causing scurvy among children. *Brit. Med. J.* Oct. 9,

322 Darroch, J. G. and Gortner, W. A. (1965). Vitamin C in canned pineapple products at the retail level. *J. Agric. Fd. Chem.* **13**, 27–29.

323 Duckworth, J. and Woodham, A. A. (1961). Leaf protein concentrates. I. Effect of source of raw material and method of drying on protein value for chicks and rats. *J. Sci. Fd. Agric.* **12**, 5–15.

324 Eheart, J. F., Young, R. W., Massey, P. H. and Havis, J. R. (1955). Crop, light intensity, soil pH and minor element effects on the yield and vitamin content of turnip greens. *Food Res.* **20**, 575–581.

325 Engst, R., Blazovich, M. and Knoll, R. (1967). Occurrence of lindane in carrots and its effects on the carotene content. *Nahrung* **11**, 389–399. (*Nutr. Abstr. Rev.* **38**, 423, 2339, 1968).

326 Ezell, B. D. and Wilcox, M. S. (1959). Loss of vitamin C in fresh vegetables as related to wilting and temperature. *J. Agric. Fd. Chem.* **7**, 507–509.

327 Ezell, B. D. and Wilcox, M. S. (1952). Influence of storage temperature on carotene, total carotenoids and ascorbic acid content of sweet potatoes. *Plant Physiol.* **27**, 81–94.

328 Ezell, B. D. and Wilcox, M. S. (1962). Loss of carotene in fresh vegetables as related to wilting and temperature. *J. Agric. Fd. Chem.* **10**, 124–126.

329 Ezell, B. D., Wilcox, M. S. and Crowder, J. N. (1952). Pre- and post-harvest changes in carotene, total carotenoids and ascorbic acid content of sweet potatoes. *Plant Physiol.* **27**, 355–369.

330 Fafunso, M. and Bassir, O. (1976). Effect of cooking on the vitamin C content of fresh leaves and wilted leaves. *J. Agric. Fd. Chem.* **24**, 354–355.

331 Fagerson, I. S., Anderson, E. E. and Hayes, K. M. (1954). Ascorbic acid content of frozen Brussels sprouts. *J. Home Econ.* **46**, 731–732.

322 Fagerson, I. S., Anderson, E. E., Hayes, K. M. and Fellers, C. R. (1954). Vitamin C and frozen strawberries. *Quick Frozen Foods* **16**, No. 9, 84–85.

333 Falconer, M. E., Fishwick, M. J., Land, D. G. and Sayer, E. R. (1964). Carotene oxidation and off-flavor development in dehydrated carrot. *J. Sci. Agric.* **15**, 897–901.

334 Fitting, K. O. and Miller, C. D. (1960). The stability of ascorbic acid in frozen and bottled acerola juice alone and combined with other fruit juices. *Food Res.* **25**, 203–210.

335 Fordham, J. R., Wells, C. E. and Chen, L. M. (1975). Sprouting of seeds and nutritional composition of seeds and sprouts. *J. Fd. Sci.* **40**, 552–556.

336 Furguson, W. E., Yates, A. R., MacQueen, K. F. and Robb, J. A. (1966). The effect of gamma-radiation on bananas. *J. Fd. Technol.* **20**, 203-205.

337 Gordon, J. and Noble, I. (1959a). Effects of blanching, freezing, freezing-storage, and cooking on ascorbic acid retention in vegetables. *J. Home Econ.* **51**, 867–870.

338 Gordon, J. and Noble, I. (1959b). Effect of cooking method on vegetables.

Ascorbic acid retention and colour difference. *J. Amer. Dietet. Assoc.* **35**, 578–581.

339 Gordon, J. and Noble, I. (1964). 'Waterless' vs boiling water cooking of vegetables. *J. Amer. Dietet. Assoc.* **44**, 378.

340 Harris, P. L. and Poland, G. L. (1939). Variations in ascorbic acid content of bananas. *Food Res.* 317–327.

341 Henshall, J. D. (1973). Fruit and vegetable products. *Proc. Nutr. Soc.* **32**, 17–22.

342 Herrmann, K., Thumann, I., Suter, G. and Nebe, G. (1973). Effect of cooking method on ascorbic acid content of kohlrabi, Brussels sprouts, cauliflower, beans and potatoes. *Ernährungs-Umschau.* **20**, 438–440. (*Fd. Sci & Technol. Abst.* 1974. 6J 814).

343 Holmes, A. D. *et al.* (1945). Vitamin content of field-frozen kale. *Am. J. Diseases Children* **70**, 298–300.

344 Holmes, A. D., Spelman, A. F. and Wetherbee, R. T. (1949). Comparison of light vs darkness for storing butternut squashes. *Food Technol.* **3**, 269–271.

345 Hoover, M. W. and Harmon, S. J. (1967). Carbohydrate changes in sweet potato flakes made by enzyme activation technique. *Food Technol.* **21**, 1529.

346 Hopp, R. J. and Merrow, S. B. (1963). Storage effects on winter squashes. Varietal differences and storage changes in the ascorbic acid content of six varieties of winter squash. *J. Agric. Fd. Chem.* **11**, 143–146.

347 Horowitz, I., Fabry, E. M. and Gerson, C. D. (1976). Bioavailability of ascorbic acid in orange juice. *J. Amer. Med. Assoc.* **235**, 2624–2625.

348 Ireson, M. G. and Eheart, M. S. (1944). Ascorbic acid losses in cooked vegetables; cooked uncovered in a large amount of water and covered in a small amount of water. *J. Home Econ.* **36**, 160–165.

349 Kalamanathan, G., Giri, J., Jaya, T. V. and Priyadarsani, P. (1974). The effect of boiling, steaming, pressure cooking and panning on the mineral and vitamin content of three vegetables. *Ind. J. Nutr. Dietet.* **11**, 10–19.

350 Kamalanathan, G., Saraswathi, G. and Devadas, R. P. (1972). Calcium, iron, thiamin and ascorbic acid content of three vegetables cooked by three methods. *Ind. J. Nutr. Dietet.* **9**, 202–205.

351 Karel, M. and Nickerson, J. T. R. (1964). Effects of relative humidity, air and vacuum on browing of dehydrated orange juice. *Food Technol.* **18**, 104.

352 Kefford, J. F. (1973). Citrus fruits and processed citrus products in human nutrition. *Wld. Rev. Nutr. Dietet.* **18**, 60–120.

353 Kefford, J. F., McKenzie, H. A. and Thompson, P. C. (1959). Effect of oxygen on quality and ascorbic acid retention in canned and frozen orange juices. *J. Sci. Fd. Agric.* **10**, 51–63.

354 Krehl, W. A. and Winters, R. W. (1950). Effect of cooking methods on retention of vitamins and minerals in vegetables. *J. Amer. Dietet. Assoc.* **26**, 966–972.

355 Krochta, J. M., Tillin, S. J. and Whitehand, L. C. (1975). Ascorbic acid content of tomatoes damaged by mechanical harvesting. *Food Technol.* **29**, 28–30; 38.

356 Kucharczyk, J., Świderski, F. *et al.* (1972). Chemical peeling of vegetables and quality and nutritive value and hygienic value of frozen vegetable products. *Nutr. Abstr. Rev.* **42**, No. 5187.

357 Lempka, A. and Prominski, W. (1967). Changes of vitamin contents of lyophilized fruits and vegetables. (*Chem. Abstr.* **67**, abstr. 63074f).

358 Malinowska, I., Mýslínka, C. and Urbánska, E. (1966–7). Factors influencing the stability of frozen fruits during freeze-storage in cold stores. *Bull. Inst. int. Froid suppl.* 409–415.

359 Mallette, M. F., Dawson, C. R., Nelson, W. L. and Gortner, W. A. (1946). Commercially dehydrated vegetables. Oxidative enzymes, vitamin content and other factors. *Ind. Eng. Chem.* **38**, 437–441.

360 McCance, R. A., Widdowson, E. M. and Shackleton, L. (1936). The nutritive value of fruits, vegetables and nuts. *Med. Res. Council Spec. Rep.* No. 213.

361 McCombs, C. L. (1957). Ascorbic acid oxidase content of certain vegetables and changes in the content of reduced and dehydro-ascorbic acid during shelf life. *Food Res.* **22**, 448–454.

362 Mizrahi, S., Labuza, T. P. and Karel, M. (1970a). Computer-aided predictions of extent of browning in dehydrated cabbage. *J. Fd. Sci.* **35**, 799–803.

363 Mizrahi, S., Labuza, T. P. and Karel, M. (1970b). Feasibility of accelerated tests for browning in dehydrated cabbage. *J. Fd. Sci.* **35**, 804–807.

364 Morgan, A. F. (1935). Nutritive value of dried fruits. *Amer. J. Public Health* **25**, 328–335.

365 Mrak, E. M. and Pfaff, H. J. (1947). Recent advances in the handling of dehydrated fruits. *Food Technol.* **1**, 147.

366 Munsell, H. E., Streightoff, F., Ben-dor, B. *et al.* (1949). Effect of large scale methods of preparation on the vitamin content of food. 3. Cabbage. *J. Amer. Dietet. Assoc.* **25**, 420–426.

367 Nelson, P. E. (1972). Processing effects on the nutritional components of horticultural crops. *Hort. Sci.* **7** (2), 151.

367a Noble, I. (1967). Effect of length of cooking. Ascorbic acid and colour of vegetables. *J. Amer. Dietet. Assoc.* **50**, 304–307.

368 Noel, G. L. and Robberstad, M. T. (1963). Stability of vitamin C in canned pineapple juice and orange juice under refrigerated conditions. *Food Technol.* **17**, 947.

369 Nutting, M. D., Neumann, H. J. and Wagner, J. R. (1970). Effect of processing variables on the stability of beta-carotene and xanthophylls of dehydrated parsley. *J. Sci. Fd. Agric.* **21**, 197–202.

370 Odland, D. and Eheart, M. S. (1975). Ascorbic acid, mineral and quality retention in frozen broccoli blanched in water, steam and ammonia-steam. *J. Fd. Sci.* **40**, 1004–1009.

371 Pantos, C. E. and Markakis, P. (1973). Ascorbic acid content of artificially ripened tomatoes. *J. Fd. Sci.* **38**, 550.

372 Pavcek, P. L. (1946). Nutritive value of dehydrated vegetables and fruits. *Ind. Eng. Chem.* **38**, 853–856.

373 Pazarinčevič-Trajkovic, J. and Baras, J. (1971). Effect of the method of drying on all-trans β-carotene in dried carrots. *Nutr. Abstr. Rev.* **41**, No. 2311.

374 Pelletier, O. and Morrison, A. B. (1965). Content and stability of ascorbic acid in fruit drinks. *J. Amer. Dietet. Assoc.* **47**, 401.

375 Purcell, A. E. (1962). Carotenoids in Goldrush sweet potato flakes. *Food Technol.* **16**(1), 99–102.

376 Rushing, N. B. and Senn, V. J. (1964). Effect of preservatives and storage temperature on shelf life of chilled citrus salads. *Food Technol.* **16**, 77–79.

377 Salunkhe, D. K. (1975). 'Storage, processing and nutritional quality of fruits and vegetables'. CRC Press, Blackwell Scientific Publications, Oxford.

378 Salunkhe, D. K., Pao, S. K. and Dull, G. G. (1973). Assessment of nutritional

value, quality and stability of cruciferous vegetables during storage and subsequent processing. *CRC Critical Reviews in Fd. Technol.* **4**, 1–38.

379   Singleton, V. L., Gortner, W. A. and Young, H. Y. (1961). Carotenoid pigments of pineapple fruit. 1. Acid-catalysed isomerisation of the pigment. *J. Fd. Sci.* **26**, 49–52.

380   Stephen, T. S. and McLemore, T. A. (1969). Preparation and storage of dehydrated carrot flakes. *Food Technol.* **23**, 1600–1602.

381   Stoll, K., Kocher, V., Gerber, H. and Bussmann, A. (1958). Studies on stored apples. *Mitt. Geb. Lebensmittel. Hyg.* **49**, 172–200.

382   Suhonen, I. (1967). Cold storage and ascorbic acid content of Brussels sprouts. *J. Sci. Agric. Soc. Finland* **39**, 99–106.

383   Sweeney, J. P. and Marsh, A. C. (1971). Effect of processing on provitamin A in vegetables. *J. Amer. Dietet. Assoc.* **59**, 238–243.

384   Thomas, P. (1975). Effect of post-harvest temperatures on quality, carotenoids and ascorbic acid content of Alphonso mangoes on ripening. *J. Fd. Sci.* **40**, 704–706.

385   Thomas, P., Dharker, S. D. and Sreenivasan, A. (1971). Effect of gamma irradiation on the post harvest physiology of five banana varieties grown in India. *J. Fd. Sci.* **36**, 243.

386   Trefether, I., Causey, K. and Fenton, F. (1951). Effect of four cooking pressures on locally grown broccoli: cooking time, palatability, ascorbic acid, thiamine and riboflavin. *Food Res.* **16**, 409–414.

387   Tressler, D. K., Moyer, J. C. and Wheeler, K. A. (1943). Losses of vitamins which may occur during the storage of dehydrated vegetables. *Amer. J. Public Health* **33**, 975–979.

388   Virgin, E. (1967). Retention of vitamin C in preparation of foods in large-scale catering. 1. Retention of vitamin C in boiling and keeping hot potatoes and vegetables. 2. Retention of vitamin C in preparation and keeping raw foods. *Int. Z. Vitaminforsch.* **37**, 10, 30.

388a   Watts, V. M. and Kik, M. C. (1947). The effects of dehydration and subsequent storage on the quality and vitamin content of vegetables. *Univ. Arkansas Agric. Exp. Sta. Bull.* **469**, 20.

389   Weckel, K. G., Santos, B., Herman, E. *et al.* (1962). Carotene components of frozen and processed carrots. *Food Technol.* **16**, 91–94.

390   Weits, J., van der Meer, M. A., Lassche, J. B. *et al.* (1970). Nutritive value and organoleptic properties of three vegetables fresh and preserved in six different ways. *Internat. Ztschr. Vitaminforsch.* **40**, 648–658.

391   Wood, M. A., Collings, A. R., Stodola, V. *et al.* (1946). Effect of large scale food preparation on vitamin retention: cabbage. *J. Amer. Dietet. Assoc.* **22**, 677–682.

392   Woodham, A. M. (1973). The effects of processing on the nutritive value of vegetable-protein concentrate. *Proc. Nutr. Soc.* **32**, 23–29.

393   Woyke, H. and Makowski, W. (1969). Vitamin C losses in deep-frozen Brussels sprouts. *Chem. Abstr.* **71**, 214, No. 11899.

394   Zscheile, F. P., Beadle, B. W. and Kraybill, H. R. (1945). Carotene content of fresh and frozen green vegetables. *Food Res.* **8**, 299–313.

See also references 513, 514, 515, 516, 519, 520, 522, 529, 530, 531, 545, 562, 569, 573, 574, 575, 577, 579, 583, 604, 611, 614, 615, 618, 624, 647, 655, 656, 664, 733, 828.

PULSES AND OILSEEDS

395 Amadi, S. C. and Hewitt, D. (1975). The digestibility and availability of lysine and methionine in isolated soya bean protein after severe heat damage. *Proc. Nutr. Soc.* **34**, 26A.

396 Anantharaman, K. and Carpenter, K. J. (1965). The effect of heat treatment on the limiting amino acids of groundnut flour for the chick. *Proc. Nutr. Soc.* **24**, xxxii.

397 Anantharaman, K. and Carpenter, K. J. (1969). Effect of heat processing on the nutritional value of groundnut products. 1. Protein quality of groundnut cotyledons for rats. *J. Sci. Fd. Agric.* **20**, 703–708.

398 Anantharaman, K. and Carpenter, K. J. (1971). Effect of heat processing on the nutritive value of groundnut products. 2. Individual amino acids. *J. Sci. Fd. Agric.* **22**, 412–418.

399 Angelo, A. J. St. and Ory, R. L. (1975). Effect of lipoperoxides on proteins in raw and processed peanuts. *J. Agric. Fd. Chem.* **23**, 141–146.

400 Arnold, J. B., Summers, J. D. and Bilanski, W. K. (1971). Nutritional value of heat treated whole soya beans. *Can. J. Anim. Sci.* **51**, 57.

401 Badenhop, A. F. and Hackler, L. R. (1971). Protein quality of dry roasted soybeans; amino acid composition and protein efficiency ratio. *J. Fd. Sci.* **36**, 1–4

402 Badenhop, A. F., Wilkins, W. F. *et al.* (1968). Roasting of soybeans as a processing technique, 53–62. Proceedings of the Symposium – 'Frontiers in Food Research'. Cornell University, N.Y. State Agric. Expt. Station, Geneva N.Y.

403 Baker, E. C. and Mustakas, G. C. (1973). Heat inactivation of trypsin inhibitor, lipoxygenase and urease in soybeans; effect of acid and base additives. *J. Amer. Oil Chem. Soc.* **50**, 137–141.

404 Bensabat, L., Frampton, V. L., Allen, L. E. and Hill, R. A. (1958). Effects of processing on the ε-amino groups of lysine in peanut proteins. *J. Agric. Fd. Chem.* **6**, 778.

405 Betschart, A. A. and Kinsella, J. E. (1974). Influence of storage on composition, amino acid content and solubility of soybean-leaf protein concentrate. *J. Agric. Fd. Chem.* **22**, 116–123.

406 Borchers, R. and Ackerson, C. W. (1950). The nutritive value of legume seeds. X. Effect of autoclaving and the trypsin inhibitor test for 17 species. *J. Nutr.* **41**, 339–345.

407 Braham, J. E., Elias, L. G. and Bressani, R. (1965). Factors affecting the nutritional quality of cottonseed meals. *J. Fd. Sci.* **30**, 531–537.

408 Bressani, R. and Elías, L. G. (1972). Nutritional Improvement of Legumes. Proc. Symp. P.A.G., Rome,

409 Bressani, R., and Elías, L. G. (1974). Legume Foods. *In* 'New Protein Foods'. Ed. A. M. Altschul. Academic Press, New York and London.

410 Buss, L. W. and Goddard, V. R. (1948). The effect of heat upon the nutritive value of peanuts. 1. Protein quality. *Food Res.* **13**, 506–511.

411 Butterworth, H. M. and Fox, H. C. (1963). The effect of heat treatment on the nutritive value of coconut meal and the prediction of nutritive value by chemical methods. *Brit. J. Nutr.* **17**, 445–452.

412 Calloway, D. H., Hickey, C. A. and Murphy, E. L. (1971). Reduction of intestinal gas-forming properties of legumes by traditional and experimental food processing methods. *J. Fd. Sci.* **36**, 251–255.

413   Daghir, N. J., Ayyash, B. and Pellett, P. L. (1969). Evaluation of groundnut meal protein for poultry. *J. Sci. Fd. Agric.* **20**, 349–354.

414   Damaty, S. M. and Hudson, B. J. F. (1975). Preparation of low-gossypol cottonseed flour. *J. Sci. Fd. Agric.* **26**, 109–115.

415   Eheart, J. F., Young, R. W. and Allison, A. H. (1955). Variety, type, year and location effect on the chemical composition of peanuts. *Food Res.* **20**, 497–505.

416   Everson, G. and Heckert, A. (1944). The biological value of some leguminous sources of protein. *J. Amer. Dietet. Assoc.* **20**, 81–82.

417   Farrell, K. T. and Fellers, C. R. (1942). Vitamin content of green snap beans. Influence of freezing, canning and dehydration on the content of thiamin, riboflavin and ascorbic acid. *Food Res.* **7**, 171–177.

418   Fenton, F., Gleime, E., Albury, M. *et al.* (1945). Effect of quantity preparation procedures on vitamin retention: canned peas. *J. Amer. Dietet. Assoc.* **21**, 700–702.

419   Fournier, S. A., Beuk, J. F., Chornock, F. W., Brown, L. C. and Rice, E. E. (1949). Determination of effect of heat on peanuts and stability of thiamine in enriched peanut butter. *Food Res.* **14**, 413–416.

420   Guerrant, N. B. and O'Hara, M. B. (1953). Vitamin retention in peas and Lima beans after blanching, freezing, processing in tin and in glass, after storage and after cooking. *Food Technol.* **7**, 473–477.

421   Hackler, L. R., Steinkraus, K. H., Van Buren, J. P. and Hand, D. B. (1964). Studies on the utilisation of tempeh protein by weanling rats. *J. Nutr.* **82**, 452-456.

422   Hackler, L. R., Van Buren, J. P., Steinkraus, K. H., El Rawi, I. and Hand, D. B. (1965). Effect of heat treatment on nutritive value of soy milk protein fed to weanling rats. *J. Fd. Sci.* **30**, 723–728.

423   Hegarty, P. V. J. and Ahn, P. C. (1976). Nutritional comparison between a soya-based meat analogue and ground beef in the unheated and heated states. *J. Fd. Sci.* **41**, 1133–1136.

424   Hesseltine, C. W. and Wang, H. L. (1972). Fermented soybean food products. *In* 'Soybeans: Chemistry and Technology', Vol. 1. Ed. Smith, A. K. and Circle, S. J. Avi Publishing Co., Westport.

425   Honavar, P. M. and Sohonie, K. (1959). Trypsin inhibitor from green gram (*Phaseolus aurens R*). *J. Sci. Indust. Res.* **18**, 202–206.

426   Jaffé, W. G. (1950). Protein digestibility and trypsin inhibitor activity of legume seeds. *Proc. Soc. Exptl. Biol. Med.* **75**, 219–220.

427   Jaffé, W. G., Moreno, R. and Wallis, V. (1973). Amylase inhibitors in legume seeds. *Nutl. Rep. Internat.* **5**, 169–174.

428   Jaffé, W. G. and Vega Lette, C. L. (1968). Heat-labile growth-inhibiting factors in beans (*Phaseolus vulgaris*). *J. Nutr.* **94**, 203–210.

429   Johnston, C. H., Schauer, L., Rapaport, S. and Deuel, H. J., Jr. (1943). The effect of cooking with and without sodium bicarbonate on the thiamine, riboflavin and ascorbic acid content of peas. *J. Nutr.* **26**, 227–239.

430   Josefsson, E. (1975). Effects of variation of heat treatment conditions on the nutritive value of low-glucosinolate rapeseed meal. *J. Sci. Fd. Agric.* **26**, 157–164; 1299–1310.

431   Kakade, M. L., Arnold, R. L., Liener, I. E. and Waibel, P. E. (1969). Unavailability of cystine from trypsin inhibitors as a factor contributing to the poor nutritive value of navy beans. *J. Nutr.* **99**, 34–42.

432   Kakade, M. L. and Evans, R. J. (1965). Growth inhibition of rats fed navy bean fractions. *J. Agric. Fd. Chem.* **13**, 450–452.

433   Kikuchi, T. (1972). Food-chemical studies on soybean and polysaccharides. III. The polysaccharides from soybeans obtained by cooking. *J. Agric. Chem. Soc. Japan* **46**, 405–409.

434   Kloe, W. De., Mantz, J. J. C. and Hartog, C. Den (1969). Nutritional aspects of textured vegetable protein. *Voeding.* **30**, 203–207. (*Food Sci. Technol. Abstr.* **1**, 1081; abstr. 9G351 1969).

435   Kon, S., Wagner, J. R. and Booth, A. N. (1974). Legume powders, preparation and some nutritional and physicochemical properties. *J. Fd. Sci.* **39**, 897–899.

436   Kylen, A. M., McCready, R. M. (1975). Nutrients in seeds and sprouts of alfalfa, lentils, mung beans and soybeans. *J. Fd. Sci.* **40**, 1008–1009.

437   Liener, I. E. (1962). Toxic factors in edible legumes and their elimination. *Amer. J. Clin. Nutr.* **11**, 281.

438   Liener, I. E. (1972). Nutritional value of food protein products. *In* 'Soybeans: Chemistry and Technology', Vol. I. Ed. Smith, A. K. and Circle, S. J. Avi Publishing Co. Inc. Westport, Conn.

439   Liener, I. E. (1976). Legume toxins in relation to protein digestibility – a review. *J. Fd. Sci.* **41**, 1076–1081.

440   Lin, K. C., Luh, B. S. and Schweigert, B. S. (1975). Folic acid content of canned Garbanzo beans. *J. Fd. Sci.* **40**, 562–565.

441   Longenecker, J. B., Martin, W. H. and Sarett, H. P. (1964). Improvement in the protein efficiency of soybean concentrates and isolates by heat treatment. *J. Agric. Fd. Chem.* **12**, 411–412.

442   Marchesini, A., Majorino, G., Montuori, F. and Cagna, D. (1975). Changes in the ascorbic and dehydroascorbic acid content of fresh and canned beans. *J. Fd. Sci.* **40**, 665–668.

443   McOsker, D. E. (1962). The limiting amino acid sequence in raw and roasted peanut protein. *J. Nutr.* **76**, 453–459.

444   Miller, C. D., Denning, H. and Bauer, A. (1952). Retention of nutrients in commercially prepared soybean curd. *Food Res.* **17**, 261–267.

445   Miller, C. F., Guadagni, D. G. and Kon, S. (1973). Vitamin retention in bean products; cooked, canned and instant bean powders. *J. Fd. Sci.* **38**, 493–495.

446   Morrison, M. H. (1974). The vitamin C and thiamin contents of quick frozen peas. *J. Fd. Technol.* **9**, 491–500.

447   Murata, K., Ikehata, H. and Miyamoto, T. (1967). Studies on the nutritional value of tempeh. *J. Fd. Sci.* **32**, 580–585.

448   Mustakas, G. C. and Griffin, E. L., Jr. (1964). Production and nutritional evaluation of extrusion-cooked full-fat soyabean flour. *J. Amer. Oil Chem. Soc.* **41**, 607–614.

449   Nene, S. P., Vakil, U. K. and Sreenivasan, A. (1975). Effects of gamma radiation on red gram (*Cajanus cajan*) proteins. *J. Fd. Sci.* **40**, 815–819.

450   Neucere, N. J., Conkerton, E. J. and Booth, A. M. (1972). Effect of heat on peanut proteins. II. Variations in nutritional quality of meals. *J. Agric. Fd. Chem.* **29**, 256.

451   Nitsan, Z. and Liener, I. E. (1976). Studies of the digestibility and retention of nitrogen and amino acids in rats fed raw and heated soy flour. *J. Nutr.* **106**, 292–299.

452   Onayemi, O. and Potter, N. N. (1976). Cowpea powders dried with methionine: preparation, storage stability, organoleptic properties, nutritional values. *J. Fd. Sci.* **41**, 48–53.

453 Phillips, M. G. and Fenton, F. (1945). Effects of home freezing and cooking on snap beans: thiamin, riboflavin, ascorbic acid. *J. Home Econ.* **37**, 164–170.

454 Powrie, W. D. and Lamberts, E. (1964). Nutritive value of proteins in canned navy beans. *Food Technol.* **18**, 111–113.

455 Quinn, M. R., Beuchat, L. R., Miller, J., Young, C. T. and Worthington, R. E. (1975). Fungal fermentation of peanut flour: effects on chemical composition and nutritive value. *J. Fd. Sci.* **40**, 470–474.

456 Raab, C. A., Luh, B. S. and Schweigert, B. S. (1973). Effect of heat processing on the retention of vitamin B_6 in Lima beans. *J. Fd. Sci.* **38**, 544–545.

457 Rackis, J. J. (1972). *In* 'Soybeans: Chemistry and Technology', Vol. 1, Proteins. Ed. Smith, A. K. and Circle, S. J. Avi Publishing Co., Westport, Conn.

458 Rao, G. R. (1974). Effect of heat on the proteins of groundnut and Bengal gram. *Ind. J. Nutr. Dietet.* **11**, 268–275.

459 Rao, M. N., Ananthachar, T. K., Kurup, K. R. *et al.* (1964). Studies on a processed protein food based on a blend of groundnut flour, and full fat soya fortified with essential amino acids, vitamins and minerals. 1. Preparation, chemical composition and shelf life. *J. Nutr. India* **1**, 1–3.

460 Rattray, E. A. S., Palmer, R. and Pusztai, A. (1974). Toxicity of kidney beans (*Phaseolus vulgaris* L.) to conventional and gnotobiotic rats. *J. Sci. Fd. Agric.* **25**, 1035–1040.

461 Rios Iriarte, B. J. and Barnes, R. H. (1966). The effect of overheating on certain nutritional properties of the protein of soybean. *Food Technol.* **20**, 835–838.

462 Robertson, J. and Sissons, D. J. (1966). The effects of maturity, processing, storage in the pod and cooking on the vitamin C content of fresh peas. *Nutrition* **20** (1), 21–27.

463 Rockland, L. B., Zaragosa, E. M., Hahn, D. M. *et al.* (1976). Retention of protein quality in quick-cooking beans prepared from dry beans. *Proc. 4th Internat. Cong. Fd. Sci. Technol.* Madrid. Vol. 1.

464 Roelofsen, P. A. and Talens, A. (1964). Changes in some B vitamins during moulding of soybeans by *Rhizopus oryzae* in the production of tempeh kedelee. *J. Fd. Sci.* **29**, 224–226.

465 Salem, S. A. (1975). Changes in carbohydrate and amino acids during baking of *Vicia faba*. *J. Sci. Fd. Agric.* **26**, 251–253.

466 Shamanthaka Sastry, M. C., Subramanian, N. and Parpia, H. A. B. (1974). Effect of dehulling and heat processing on nutritional value of sesame proteins. *J. Amer. Oil Chem. Soc.* **51**, 115–118.

467 Shemer, M. and Perkins, E. G. (1975). Degradation of methionine in heated soybean protein and the formation of β-methylmercapto-propionaldehyde. *J. Agric. Fd. Chem.* **23**, 201–204.

468 Shemer, M. Wei, L. S. and Perkins, E. G. (1973). Nutritional and chemical studies of three processed soybean foods. *J. Fd. Sci.* **38**, 112–115.

469 Skurray, G. R. and Osborne, C. (1976). Nutritional value of soya protein and milk coprecipitates in sausage products. *J. Sci. Fd. Agric.* **27**, 175–180.

470 Tauber, H., Kershaw, B. B. and Wright, R. D. (1949). Studies on the growth inhibitor fractions of Lima beans and isolation of a crystalline heat-stable inhibitor. *J. biol. Chem.* **179**, 1155–1161.

471 Valledevi, A., Ramanuja, M. N., Rao, N. A. N. and Nath, H. (1972). Effects of processing and storage on thiamin, riboflavin and nicotinic acid contents of four varieties of Indian pulses. *Ind. J. Nutr. Dietet.* **9**, 336–341.

472   Van Buren, J. P., Steinkraus, K. H., Hackler, L. R. *et al.* (1964). Indices of protein quality in dried soymilk. *J. Agric. Fd. Chem.* **12**, 524–527.
473   Van Veen, A. G., Hackler, L. R., Steinkraus, K. H. and Mukherjee, S. K. (1967). Nutritive quality of Idli, a fermented food of India. *J. Fd. Sci.* **32**, 339–341.
474   Varela, G., Vidal, C. and Zamora, S. (1970). Effect of heat treatment on the content of amino acids and available lysine in groundnut protein. *Ann. de Bromatologia* **22**, 323–329.
475   Wu, C. H. and Fenton, F. (1953). Effect of sprouting and cooking of soybeans on palatability, lysine, tryptophan, thiamine and ascorbic acid. *Food Res.* **18**, 640–645.
476   Ziprin, Y. A. and Carlin, A. F. (1976), microwave and conventional cooking in relation to quality and nutritive value of beef and beef-soy loaves. *J. Fd. Sci.* **41**, 4–8.

See also references 517, 518, 520, 521, 528, 579, 596, 616, 617, 630, 633, 634, 635, 636, 658A, 750, 779A, 779B, 835, 840, 885.

POTATOES

477   Augustin, J. (1975). Variations in the nutritional composition of fresh potatoes. *J. Fd. Sci.* **40**, 1295–1299.
478   Augustin, J., McDole, R. E., McMaster, D. M. *et al.* (1975). Ascorbic acid in Russet Burbank potatoes. *J. Fd. Sci.* **40**, 415–416.
479   Bring, S. V., Grassl, C., Hofstrand, J. T. and Willard, M. J. (1963). Total ascorbic acid in potatoes. *J. Amer. Dietet. Assoc.* **42**, 320–324.
480   Cording, J., Jr., Eskew, R. K., Salinard, G. J. and Sullivan, J. F. (1961). Vitamin stability in fortified potato flakes. *Food Technol.* **15**, 279–282.
481   Domah, A. A. M. B., Davidek, J. and Velisek, J. (1974). Changes of L-ascorbic and L-dehydroascorbic acids during cooking and frying of potatoes. *Food Sci. Technol. Abstr.* **9J**, 1337.
482   Eddy, T. P. and Stock, A. (1972). Losses of vitamin C during machine peeling and soaking of peeled potatoes. *Proc. Nutr. Soc.* **31**, 87A–88A.
483   Fujimaki, M., Makoto, T. and Matsumoto, T. (1968). Effect of gamma-irradiation on the amino acids of potatoes. *Agric. Biol. Chem.* **32**, 1228–1231.
484   Gleim, E., Albury, M., McCartney, J. R. *et al.* (1946a). Ascorbic acid, thiamine, riboflavin, and niacin content of potatoes in large-scale food service. *Food Res.* **11**, 461.
485   Hanning, F. and Mudambi, S. R. (1962). Dehydrated and canned potatoes. Thiamine and biologically active ascorbic acid. *J. Amer. Dietet. Assoc.* **40**, 211–213.
486   Hendel, C. E., Silveira, V. and Harrington, W. O. (1955). Rates of nonenzymatic browning of white potatoes during dehydration. *Food Technol.* **9**, 433–438.
487   Hawkins, W. W., Leonard, V. G. and Armstrong, J. E. (1961). Effectiveness of ascorbic acid in preventing the darkening of oil-blanched French-fried potatoes. *Food Technol.* **15**, 410.
488   Jadhav, S., Steele, L. and Hadzlyev, D. (1975). Vitamin C losses during production of dehydrated mashed potatoes. *Lebensmittel-Wissenschaft-u. Technol.* **8**, 225.
488a Mapson, L. W. and Wager, H. G. (1961). Preservation of peeled potatoes. I. Use of sulphite and its effect on thiamine content. *J. Sci. Fd. Agric.* **12**, 43–49.

489   Melnick, D. (1957). Investigated potato chip factors. *J. Amer. Oil Chem. Soc.* **34**, 351.
490   Mudambi, S. R. and Hanning, F. (1962). Effect of sulphiting on potatoes. Acceptability and thiamine and ascorbic acid content. *J. Amer. Dietet. Assoc.* **40**, 214–217.
491   Myers, P. W. and Roehm, G. H. (1963). Ascorbic acid in dehydrated potatoes. *J. Amer. Dietet. Assoc.* **42**, 325–327.
492   Oguntona, T. E. and Bender, A. E. (1976). Loss of thiamin from potatoes. *J. Fd. Technol.* **11**, 347–352.
493   Page, E. and Hanning, F. M. (1963). Retention after storage and cooking of vitamin B_6 and niacin in potatoes. *J. Amer. Dietet. Assoc.* **42**, 42–45.
494   Somogyi, J. C., Trautner, K. and Kopp, P. (1971). Importance of potato products in todays diet. *Bibliotheca Nutritio et dieta* **16**, 140–154.
495   Sullivan, J. F., *et al.* (1974). Flavour and storage stability of explosion-puffed potatoes: non-enzymatic browning. *J. Fd. Sci.* **39**, 58–60.
496   Streightoff, F., Munsell, H. E., Ben-dor, B. *et al.* (1946). Effect of large-scale methods of preparation on vitamin content of food. 1. Potatoes. *J. Amer. Dietet. Assoc.* **22**, 117–127.
497   Wertz, A. W. and Weir, C. E. (1964). Effect of institutional cooking methods on vitamin content of foods. 2. Ascorbic acid content of potatoes. *Food Res.* **11**, 319.
498   Winterton, D. (1969). Potato crisp quality. The effect of nitrogen fertilizer application. *Food Sci. Technol. Abstr.* **1**, 998; abstr. 8J698.
499   Witkowski, C. and Paradowski, A. (1976). Effect of the time and temperature of sterilisation on vitamin C in canned potatoes. *Nutr. Abst. Rev.* **46**, No. 5031.
500   Zarnegar, L. and Bender, A. E. (1971). The stability of vitamin C in machine-peeled potatoes. *Proc. Nutr. Soc.* **30**, 94A.

EGGS

501   Coppock, J. B. M. and Daniels, N. W. R. (1962). Influence of diet and husbandry on the nutritional value of the hen's egg. *J. Sci. Fd. Agric.* **13**, 459–469.
502   Denton, C. A., Cabell, C. A., Bastron, H. and Davis, R. (1944). The effect of spray drying and the subsequent storage of the dried product on the vitamins A, D and riboflavin content of eggs. *J. Nutr.* **28**, 421–426.
503   Evans, R. J., Bandemer, S. L. and Butts, H. A. (1949). The amino acid content of fresh and stored shell eggs. *J. Poultry Sci.* **28**, 697–702.
504   Evans, R. J., Davidson, J. A. and Butts, H. A. (1949). Changes in egg proteins occurring during cold storage of shell eggs. *J. Poultry Sci.* **28**, 206–214.
505   Evans, R. J. *et al.* (1951–53). The niacin (riboflavin, choline, biotin) content of fresh and stored shell eggs. *J. Poultry Sci.* **30**, 132–135; **31**, 269–273; **30**, 29–33; **32**, 680–683.
506   Evans, R. J., Davidson, J. A., Bauer, D. and Butts, H. A. (1953). Folic acid in fresh and stored shell eggs. *J. Agric. Fd. Chem.* **1**, 170–172.
507   Everson, G. J., Souders, H. J. (1957). Composition and nutritive importance of eggs. *J. Amer. Dietet. Assoc.* **33**, 1244–1254.
508   Hauge, S. M. and Zscheile, F. P. (1942). The effect of dehydration upon the vitamin A content of eggs. *Science* **96**, 536.

509 Hawthorne, J. R. and Brooks, J. (1944). Dried egg. VIII. Removal of the sugar of egg pulp before drying. A method of improving the storage life of spray-dried whole egg. *J. Soc. Chem. Ind.* **63**, 232–234.

510 Klose, A. A., Jones, G. I. and Fevold, H. L. (1943). Vitamin content of spray-dried whole egg. *Ind. Eng. Chem.* **35**, 1203–1205.

511 Tolan, A., Robertson, J., Orton, C. R., Head, M. J. *et al.* (1974). Studies on the composition of food. 5. The chemical composition of eggs produced under battery, deep litter and free range conditions. *Brit. J. Nutr.* **31**, 185–200.

512 Whitford, C., Pickering, C., Summers, K., Weis, A. and Bisbey, B. (1951). The vitamin content of eggs as affected by dehydration and storage. *Univ. Missouri Agr. Expt. Sta. Res. Bull.* No. 483, 12.

PROCESSING METHODS
Blanching

513 Adam, W. B., Horner, G. and Stanworth, J. (1942). Changes occurring in blanching of vegetables. *J. Soc. Chem. Ind. London* **61**, 96–99.

514 Bomben, J. L., Dietrich, W. C., Hudson, J. S. *et al.* (1975). Yields and solids loss in steam blanching, cooling and freezing vegetables. *J. Fd. Sci.* **40**, 660–664.

515 Dietrich, W. C., Huxsell, C. C. and Guadagni, D. G. (1970). Comparison of microwave, conventional and combination blanching of Brussels sprouts for frozen storage. *Food Technol.* **24**, 613–617.

516 Eheart, M. S. (1967). Effect of microwave versus water-blanching on nutrients in broccoli. *J. Amer. Dietet. Assoc.* **50**, 207–211.

517 Feaster, J. F., Mudra, A. E., Ives, M. and Tompkins, M. D. (1949). Effect of blanching time on vitamin retention in canned peas. *Canner* **108**, No. 1, 27–30.

518 Guerrant, N. B. and Dutcher, R. A. (1948). Further observations concerning the relationship of temperature of blanching to ascorbic acid retention in green beans. *Arch. Biochem.* **18**, 353–359.

519 Guerrant, N. B., Vavitch, M. G., Fardig, O. B. *et al.* (1947). Effect of duration and temperature of blanch on vitamin retention by certain vegetables. *Ind. Eng. Chem.* **39**, 1000–1007.

520 Hard, M. M. and Ross, E. (1956). Dielectric scalding of spinach, peas and snap beans for freezing preservation. *Food Technol.* **10**, 241–244.

521 Holmquist, J. W., Clifcorn, L. E., Heberlein, D. G. and Schmidt, C. F. (1954). Steam blanching of peas. *Food Technol.* **8**, 437–445.

522 Hudson, M. A., Sharples, V. J. *et al.* (1974). Quality of home frozen vegetables: I. Effects of blanching and/or cooling in various solutions on organoleptic assessments and vitamin C content. *J. Fd. Technol.* **9**, 95–103.

523 Lazar, N. E., Lund, D. B. and Dietrich, W. C. (1971). A new concept in blanching. (IQB). *Food Technol.* **25**, 684–686.

524 Lea, F. A. (1958). The blanching process. *Adv. Fd. Res.* **8**, 63–109.

525 Lund, D. B. (1975). Effects of blanching, pasteurisation and sterilisation on nutrients. *In* 'Nutritional Evaluation of Food Processing', 205–240. Ed. Harris, R. S. and Karmas, E. Avi Publishing Co., Westport, Conn.

526 Lund, D. B., Bruin, S. Jr. and Lazar, M. E. (1972). Internal temperature distribution during individual quick blanching. *J. Fd. Sci.* **37**, 167.

527 Melnick, D., Hochberg, M. and Oser, B. L. (1944). Comparative study of steam and hot water blanching. *Food Res.* **9**, 148–153.
528 Mitchell, R. S., Board, P. W. and Lynch, L. J. (1968). Fluidized-bed blanching of green peas for processing. *Food Technol.* **22**, 717–718.
529 Moyer, J. C. and Stotz, E. (1947). The blanching of vegetables by electronics. *Food Technol.* **1**, 252–257.
530 Noble, I. and Gordon, J. (1964). Effect of blanching method on ascorbic acid and colour of frozen vegetables. *J. Amer. Dietet. Assoc.* **44**, 120–123.
531 Ralls, J. W., Maagdenberg, H. J., Yacoub, N. L. *et al.* (1973). In plant, continuous hot-gas blanching of spinach. *J. Fd. Sci.* **38**, 192–194.

See also references 337, 370.

Drying

532 Bluestein, P. M. and Labuza, T. P. (1975). Effect of moisture removal on nutrients. *In* 'Nutritional Evaluation of Food Processing', 289–323. Ed. Harris, R. S. and Karmas, E. Avi publishing Co., Westport, Conn.
533 De Groot, A. P. (1963). The influence of dehydration of foods on the digestibility and the biological value of the protein. *Food Technol.* **17**, 339–343.
534 Della Monica, E. S. and McDowell, P. E. (1965). Comparison of β-carotene content of dried carrot prepared by three dehydration processes. *Food Technol.* **19**, 141–143.
535 Goldblith, S. A. and Tannenbaum, S. R. (1966). The nutritional aspects of the freeze drying of foods. *Proc. 7th Internat. Cong. Nutr.*, Vol. 4. Vieweg and Son, Hamburg, Germany.
536 Goodling, E. G. B. (1962). The storage behaviour of dehydrated foods. *In* 'Recent Advances in Food Science', Vol. 2. Ed. Leitch, J. M. and Hawthorn, J. Butterworths, London.
537 Holdsworth, S. D. (1971). Dehydration of food products. *Food Technol.* **6**, 331–370.
538 Hollingsworth, D. F. (1961). Nutritive value. *In* 'The Accelerated Freeze-drying Method of Food Preservation', Chap. XIII, 132–137. Ministry of Agriculture, Fisheries and Food. HMSO, London.
538a Kaufman, V. F., Wong, F. M., Taylor, D. H. and Talburt, W. F. (1955). Problems in the production of tomato juice powder by vacuum. *Food Technol.* **9**, 120.
539 Labuza, T. P. (1972). Nutrient losses during drying and storage of dehydrated foods. CRC Critical Reviews of Food Technology, **3**, 217–240.
540 Labuza, T. P. (1973). Effects of dehydration and storage. *Food Technol.* **27**, 20–26.
541 Lea, C. H. (1958). Fundamental aspects of the dehydration of food. Soc. Chem. Ind. Monograph.
542 Livingston, A. L., Allis, M. E. and Kobler, G. O. (1971). Amino acid stability during alfalfa dehydration. *J. Agric. Fd. Chem.* **19**, 947–950.
543 Loncin, M., Bimbenet, J. J. and Lenges, J. (1968). Influence of the activity of water on spoilage of foodstuffs. *J. Fd. Technol.* **3**, 131–142.
544 Mills, R. C. and Hart, E. B. (1945). Studies on the stabilization of carotene in dehydrated foods and feeds. *J. Dairy Sci.* **28**, 1–13.

545 Morgan, A. F., Carl, B. C., Hunner, M. C. *et al.* (1944). Vitamin losses in commercially produced dehydrated vegetables; cabbage, potatoes, carrots and onions. *Fruit Prod. J.* **23**, 207–211.
546 Rice, E. E., Beuk, J. F., Kauffman, F. L. *et al.* (1944). Preliminary studies on the stabilization of thiamine in dehydrated foods. *Food Res.* **9**, 491–499.
547 Thomas, M. H. and Calloway, D. H. (1961). Nutritional value of dehydrated foods. *J. Amer. Dietet. Assoc.* **39**, 105–116.
548 Von Loesecke, H. W. (1955). 'Drying and Dehydration of Foods'. Reinhold Publishing Corp., New York.

See also references, 77, 81, 86.

Canning

549 Cameron, E. J. (1954). The canning industry nutrition program. *Food Technol.* **8**, 586–592.
550 Cameron, E. J. (1955). Retention of Nutrients during Canning. National Canners Assoc. Washington, DC.
551 Cameron, E. J., Clifcorn, L. E., Esty, J. R. *et al.* (1955). 'Retention of Nutrients during Canning', Res. Lab. Nat. Canners Assoc. U.S.A.
552 Cameron, E. J., Pilcher, R. W. and Clifcorn, L. E. (1949). Nutrient retention during canned food production. *Amer. J. Pub. Health* **39**, 756–763.
553 Cecil, S. R. and Woodroof, J. G. (1963). The stability of canned foods in long-term storage. *Food Technol.* **17** (5), 131.
554 Everson, G. J., Chang, J., Leonard, S., Luh, B. S. and Simone, M. (1964). Aseptic canning of foods. II. Thiamine retention as influenced by processing method, storage time and temperature, and type of container. III. Pyridoxine. *Food Technol.* **18**, 84–86; 87–88.
555 Farrow, R. P., Lamb, F. C., Elkins, E. R., Low, N., Humphrey, J. and Kemper, K. (1973). Nutritive content of canned tomato juice and whole kernel corn. *J. Fd. Sci.* **38**, 593–601.
556 Freed, M., Brenner, S. and Wodicka, V. O. (1949). Prediction of thiamin and ascorbic acid stability in stored canned foods. *Food Technol.* **3**, 148–151.
557 Guerrant, N. B., Fardig, O. B., Vavich, M. G. and Ellenberger, H. E. (1948). Nutritive value of canned food. Influence of temperature and time of storage on vitamin content. *Ind. Eng. Chem.* **40**, 2258–2263.
558 Guerrant, N. B., Vavich, M. G. and Dutcher, R. A. (1945). Nutritive value of canned foods. Influence of temperature and time of storage on vitamin contents. *Ind. Eng. Chem.* **37**, 1240–1243.
559 Hayakawa, K. (1969). New parameters for calculating mass average sterilizing value to estimate nutrients in thermally conductive foods. *Can. Inst. Fd. Technol. J.* **2**, 165.
560 Hellendoorn, E. W., de Groot, A. P., Slump, P. *et al.* (1969). Effect of sterilisation and three years; storage on the nutritive value of canned prepared meals. *Voeding* **30**, 44–63. (*Food Sci. Technol. Abstr.* **1**, 967; abstr. 8G333, 1969).
561 Henshall, J. D. (1974). Vitamin C in canning and freezing. *In* 'Vitamin C'. Ed. Birch, G. G. and Parker, K. J. Applied Science Publishers, London.
562 Hinman, W. F., Brush, M. K. and Halliday, F. G. (1944). The nutritive value of canned foods. 6. Effect of large scale preparation for serving on the ascorbic

acid, thiamine and riboflavin content of commercially-canned vegetables. *J. Amer. Dietet. Assoc.* **20**, 752.

563 Hinman, W. F., Higgins, M. M. and Halliday, E. G. (1947). The nutritive value of canned foods. 18. Further studies on carotene, ascorbic acid and thiamine. *J. Amer. Dietet. Assoc.* **23**, 226–231.

564 Ingalls, R., Brewer, W. D., Tobey, H. L., Plummer, J. *et al.* (1950). Nutritive value of canned foods. *Food Technol.* **4**, 258–263, 264.

565 Ives, M., Wagner, J. R., Elvehjem, C. A. and Strong, F. M. (1944). The nutritive value of canned foods. 3. Thiamin and niacin. *J. Nutr.* 117–121.

566 Kramer, A. (1946). Nutritive value of canned foods. 61. Proximate and mineral composition. *Food Res.* **11**, 391–398.

567 Monroe, K. H., Brighton, K. W. and Bendix, G. H. (1949). The nutritive value of canned foods. 28. Some studies of commercial warehouse temperatures with reference to the stability of vitamins in canned foods. *Food Technol.* **3**, 292–299.

568 Pressley, A., Ridder, C., Smith, M. C. and Caldwell, E. (1944). Nutritive value of canned foods. 2. Ascorbic acid and carotene and vitamin A content. *J. Nutr.* **28**, 107.

569 Sheft, B. B., Griswold, R. M. *et al.* (1949). Nutritive value of canned foods. Effect of time and temperature of storage on vitamin content of commercial canned fruits and fruit juices (stored 18 and 24 months). *Ind. Eng. Chem.* **41**, 144–145.

570 Svabova-Stronova, M. (1968). Changes in the biological value of proteins in canned foods. *Chem. Abstr.* **70**, abstr. 18981, 1969.

571 Tepley, L. J., Derse, P. H. and Krieger, C. (1953). Nutritive value of canned foods. Vitamin B_6, folic acid, β-carotene, ascorbic acid, thiamine, riboflavin and niacin content and proximate composition. *J. Agric. Fd. Chem.* **1**, 1204–1207.

572 Thompson, M. L., Cunningham, E. and Snell, E. E. (1944). The nutritive value of canned foods. 4. Riboflavin and pantothenic acid. *J. Nutr.* **28**, 123–129.

573 Wagner, J. R., Strong, F. M. and Elvehjem, C. A. (1947). Nutritive value of canned foods. Effect of blanching on the retentions of ascorbic acid, thiamine and niacin in vegetables. *Ind. Eng. Chem.* **39**, 985–990; 990–993.

See also references 4, 58, 77, 79, 417, 418, 440, 442, 485.

Freezing

574 Ang, C. Y. W., Chang, C. M., Frey, A. E. and Livingstone, G. E. (1975). Effect of heating methods on vitamin retention in six fresh and frozen prepared food products. *J. Fd. Sci.* **40**, 997–1003.

575 Causey, K. and Fenton, F. (1951). Effect of reheating on palatability, nutritive value and bacterial count of frozen cooked foods. I. Vegetables. *J. Amer. Dietet. Assoc.* **27**, 390–395.

576 Causey, K. and Fenton, F. (1951b). Effect of reheating on palatability, nutritive value and bacterial count of frozen cooked foods. II. Meat dishes. *J. Amer. Dietet. Assoc.* **27**, 491–495.

577 Clegg, K. M. (1974). Frozen vegetables. *Nutrition and Food Sci.* **36**, 6–8.

578 De Ritter, E., Osadca, M., Scheiner, J. and Keating, J. (1974). Vitamins in frozen convenience dinners and pot pies. *J. Amer. Dietet. Assoc.* **64**, 391–397.

579 Derse, P. H. and Teply, L. J. (1958). Effect of storage conditions on nutrients in frozen green beans, peas, orange juice and strawberries. *J. Agric. Fd. Chem.* **6**, 309–312.

580 Eddy, T. P., Nicholson, A. L. and Wheeler, E. F. (1968). Precooked frozen foods; The effects of heating on vitamin C. *Nutrition, Lond.* **22**, 122–128.

581 Fennema, O. (1975). Effects of freeze-preservation on nutrients. *In* 'Nutritional Evaluation of Food Processing', 244–288. Ed. Harris, R. S. and Karmas, E. Avi Publishing Co., Westport, Conn.

582 Gleim, S. A. and Fenton, F. (1949). Effects of 0°F and 15°F storage on the quality of frozen cooked foods. *Food Technol.* **3**, 187–192.

583 Gleim, E. G., Tressler, D. K. and Fenton, F. (1944). Ascorbic acid, thiamin, riboflavin and carotene contents of asparagus and spinach in the fresh, stored and frozen states, both before and after cooking. *Food Res.* **9**, 471–490.

584 Hoppner, K., Lampi, B. and Perrin, D. E. (1973). Folacin activity of frozen convenience foods. *J. Amer. Dietet. Assoc.* **63**, 536–539.

585 Hucker, G. J. and Clarke, A. (1961). Effect of alternate freezing and thawing on the ascorbic acid content of frozen vegetables. *Food Technol.* **15**, 50–51.

586 International Institute of Refrigeration (1971). Recommendations for the Processing and Handling of Frozen Foods, 2nd Ed. International Inst. of Refrigeration, Paris.

587 Kahn, L. N. and Livingstone, G. E. (1970). Effect of heating methods on thiamin retention in fresh or frozen prepared foods. *J. Fd. Sci.* **35**, 349–351.

588 Kemp, G. (1970). Developments in frozen foods. *Agriculture* **77**, 9–12.

589 Van Arsdel, W. B. (1957). The time-temperature tolerance of frozen foods. 1. Introduction – the problem and attack. *Food Technol.* **11**, 28–33.

590 Van Arsdel, W. B., Copley, M. J. and Olsen, R. L. (1969). 'Quality and Stability of Frozen foods. Time-temperature Tolerance and its Significance'. Wiley-Interscience, New York.

591 Watt, B. K. (1968). Nutritive value of frozen foods. *In* 'The Freezing Preservation of Foods', 4th Edn., Vol. 2, Ed. Tressler, D. K., Van Arsdel, W. B. and Copley, M. J. Avi Publishing Co., Westport, Conn.

See also references 9, 13, 27, 49, 50, 52, 53, 61, 74, 75, 101, 331, 332, 337, 343, 370, 417, 446, 453, 514, 515, 605, 664.

OTHER PROCESSING METHODS

592 Apger, J., Cox, N., Downey, I. and Fenton, F. (1959). Cooking pork electronically. Effect on cooking time, losses and quality. *J. Amer. Dietet. Assoc.* **35**, 1260–1269.

593 Aref, M. M. *et al.* (1972). Inactivation of α-amylase in wheat flour with microwaves. *J. Microwave Power* **7** (3), 215–221.

594 Beetner, G., Tsao, T., Frey, A. and Harper, J. (1974). Degradation of thiamin and riboflavin during extrusion processing. *J. Fd. Sci.* **39**, 207–208.

595 Besser, T. and Kramer, A. (1972). Changes in quality and nutritional composition of foods preserved by gas exchange. *J. Fd. Sci.* **37**, 820–823.

596 Borchers, R., Manage, L. D., Nelson, S. O. and Stetson, L. E. (1972). Rapid improvement in nutritional quality of soybeans by dielectric heating. *J. Fd. Sci.* **37**, 333–334.

597　Bowers, J. A. *et al.* (1974). Turkey cooked in microwave and conventional ovens. *Poultry Sci.* **53**, 844.

598　Bowers, J. A., Fryer, B. A. and Engler, P. P. (1974). Vitamin B_6 in pork muscle cooked in microwave and conventional ovens. *J. Fd. Sci.* **39**, 426–427.

599　Bowman, T. P. *et al.* (1975). Vegetables cooked by microwave versus conventional methods. Retention of reduced ascorbic acid and chlorophyll. *Microwave Energy Applic. Newsl.* **8** (3), 3–8.

600　Brubacher, G., Bernhard, G. and Ritzel, G. (1972). Vitamin content of meals prepared in cooking automats. *Nutr. Abstr. Rev.* **40**, No. 7167. (In German.)

601　Campbell, C. L., Lin, T. Y. and Proctor, B. E. (1958). Microwave versus conventional cooking. *J. Amer. Dietet. Assoc.* **34**, 365–370.

602　Clegg, K. M. and Lewis, S. E. (1963). The vitamin B content of foodstuffs fumigated with methyl bromide. *J. Sci. Fd. Agric.* **14**, 548–552.

603　Daun, H. (1975). Effects of salting, curing and smoking on nutrients in flesh foods. *In* 'Nutritional Evaluation of Food Processing', 355–381. Ed. Harris, R. S. and Karmas, E. Avi Publishing Co., Westport, Conn.

604　Dennison, R. A. and Ahmed, E. M. (1971–1972). Effects of low level irradiation on the preservation of fruits: a 7 year summary. *Isotopes radiation Technol.* **9**, 194–200.

605　Eddy, T. P., Nicholson, A. L. and Wheeler, E. F. (1969). Precooked frozen foods: 2. The use of microwave ovens. *Nutrition, Lond.* **23**, 14–22.

606　Eheart, M. S. and Gott, C. (1965). Chlorophyll, ascorbic acid and pH changes in green vegetables cooked by stir-fry, microwave and conventional methods. *Food Technol.* **19**, 867–870.

606a　Faizur Rahman, A. T. M. (1975). Radiation research in Bangladesh. *Food Irradiation Information* **4**, 6.

607　FAO (1968). Report of the FAO Technical Conference on the Freezing and Irradiation of Fish, organised jointly with the International Institute of Refrigeration and the International Atomic Energy Agency. Madrid 1967. UN Food and Agriculture Organisation Fisheries Report No. 53. FAO, Rome.

608　Ford, J. E., Gregory, M. E. and Thompson, S. Y. (1962). Liquid milk. Effect of gamma-irradiation on vitamins and proteins. 16th International Dairy Congress. Copenhagen, Vol. A. p. 917.

609　Goldblith, S. A. (1970). Radiation preservation of food. The current status. *J. Fd. Technol.* **5**, 103–110.

610　Goldblith, S. A. and Proctor, B. E. (1949). Effect of high-voltage X-rays and cathode rays on vitamins (riboflavin and carotene). *Nucleonics* **5**, 50–58.

611　Gordon, J. and Noble, I. (1959). Comparison of electronic versus conventional cooking of vegetables. Flavour, colour and ascorbic acid retention. *J. Amer. Dietet. Assoc.* **35**, 241–244.

612　Gounelle, H., Gulat-Marnay, C. and Fauchet, M. (1970). Effects of ionising irradiation on the vitamins B and C contents of food. *Ann. Nutr. Aliment.* **24**, 41–49.

613　Groninger, H. S. and Tappel, A. L. (1957). The destruction of thiamine in meats and in aqueous solution by gamma radiation. *Food Res.* **22**, 519–523.

613a　Guesseri, G. (1975). Radiation sources and dosimetry in Italy. *Food Irradiation Information* **4**, 33.

614　Harris, R. S. and Mosher, L. M. (1941). Effect of reduced evaporation on the provitamin A content of lettuce in refrigerated storage. *Food Res.* **6**, 387.

615　Harris, R. S., Wissman, H. B. and Greenlie, D. (1940). The effect of reduced evaporation on the vitamin content of fresh vegetables in refrigerated storage. *J. Lab. Clin. Med.* **25**, 838–843.

616 Hutton, K. and Foxcroft, P. D. (1974). Effect of processing temperature on some parameters of nutritional significance for micronized soya beans. *Proc. Nutr. Soc.* **34**, 49A.

617 Hutton, K. and Thompson, A. (1975). Effect of micronizing on the utilisation of soya beans by growing rats. *Proc. Nutr. Soc.* **34**, 50A.

618 Janave, M. T. (1973). Polyphenol oxidase activity and browning of mango fruit induced by gamma irradiation. *J. Fd. Sci.* **38**, 149.

619 Jones, I. D. (1975). Effects of processing by fermentation on nutrients. *In* 'Nutritional Evaluation of Food Processing', 324–354. Ed. Harris, R. S. and Karmas, E. Avi Publishing Co., Westport, Conn.

620 Josephson, E. S., Thomas, M. H. and Calhoun, W. K. (1975). Effects of treatment of foods with ionising radiation. *In* 'Nutritional Evaluation of Food Processing'. Ed. Harris, R. S. and Karmas, E. Avi Publishing Co., Westport, Conn.

621 Keay, J. N. (1968). The effect of doses of gamma radiation up to 16 Mrads. on plastic packaging materials for fish. *J. Fd. Technol.* **3**, 123–129.

622 Kennedy, T. S. (1965). Nutritional value of foods treated with gamma radiation. 1. Effects on some B-complex vitamins in egg and wheat. *J. Sci. Fd. Agric.* **16**, 81–84 ; 433–437.

623 Kung, H., Gaden, E. L. and King, C. G. (1953). Vitamins and enzymes in milk. Effect of gamma radiation on activity. *J. Agric. Fd. Chem.* **1**, 142–144.

624 Kylen, A. M., Charles, V. R., McGrath, B. H. *et al.* (1961). Microwave cooking of vegetables. Ascorbic acid retention and palatability. *J. Amer. Dietet. Assoc.* **39**, 321–326.

625 Kylen, A. M., McGrath, B. H., Hallmark, E. L. and Van Duyne, F. O. (1964). Microwave and conventional cooking of meat. *J. Amer. Dietet. Assoc.* **45**, 139.

626 Lawrence, T. L. J. (1973). An evaluation of the micronisation process for preparing cereals for the growing pig. *Animal Prod.* **16**, 99–107 ; 109–116.

627 Labuza, T. P. (1976). Intermediate moisture foods; chemical and nutrient stability. *Proc. 4th Internat. Cong. Fd. Sci. Technol.* Madrid. Vol. 1.

628 Labuza, T. P., Tannenbaum, S. R. and Karel, M. (1970). Water content and stability of low-moisture and intermediate-moisture foods. *Food Technol.* **24**, 543–550.

629 Livingston, G. E., Ang, C. Y. W. and Chang, C. M. (1973). Effect of food service handling. *Food Technol.* **27**, 28–34.

630 Lotti, G., Anelli, G., LoMoro, A. and Teglio, A. (1975). Effect of gamma-irradiation on the proteins of leguminous seeds. *Food Sci. Tech. Abst.* **5G**, 249.

631 Manson, J. E., Zahradnik, J. W. and Stumbo, C. R. (1970). Evaluation of lethality and nutrient retentions of conduction-heating foods in rectangular containers. *Food Technol.* **24**, 1297–1301.

632 McMillan, P. (1968). Microwave cooking. A review of the literature reporting comparison between food cooked in microwave ovens and by conventional methods. *Rev. Nutr. Food Sci.* 13–16.

633 McNab, J. M. and Wilson, B. J. (1974). Effects of micronising on the utilisation of Field Beans (*Vicia faba* L.) by the young chick. *J. Sci. Fd. Agric.* **25**, 395–400.

634 Muelenaere, H. J. H. de, and Buzzard, J. L. (1969). Cooker extruders in service of world feeding. *Food Technol.* **23**, 345–351.

635 Mustakas, G. C., Griffin, E. L., Allen, L. E. and Smith, O. B. (1964). Production and nutritional evaluation of extrusion-cooked full-fat soybean flour. *J. Amer. Oil Chem. Soc.* **41**, 607.

636 Mustakas, G. C., Albrecht, W. J., Bookwalter, G. N. *et al.* (1970). Extruder-processing to improve nutritional quality; flavour and keeping quality of full-fat soy flour. *Food Technol.* **24**, 1290–1296.

637 Neal, W. T. L. (1964). Prospects for radiation preservation of foods in Britain. *Proc. Int. Conf. Radiation Preserv. Foods, Boston, Mass.* Nat. Acad. Sci., Nat. Res. Counc. Publ. No. 127.

638 Noble, I. and Gomez, L. (1962). Vitamin retention in meat cooked electronically. Thiamine and riboflavin in lamb and bacon. *J. Amer. Dietet. Assoc.* **41**, 217–270.

639 Platt, B. S. (1964). Biological ennoblement: improvement of the nutritive value of foods and dietary regimens by biological agencies. *Food Technol.* **18**, No. 5, 68-76.

640 Proctor, B. E. and Goldblith, S. A. (1948). Radar energy for rapid food cooking and blanching and its effect on vitamin content. *Food Technol.* **2**, 95.

641 Proctor, B. E. and Goldblith, S. A. (1949). Effect of soft X-rays on vitamins (niacin, riboflavin and ascorbic acid). *Nucleonics* **5**, 56–62.

642 Proctor, B. E., Nickerson, J. T. R. and Licciardello, J. J. (1956). Cathode ray irradiation of chicken meat for the extension of shelf life. *Food Res.* **21**, 11–20.

643 Putnam, M. (1973). Micronisation – a new feed processing technique. *J. Flour and Animal Feed Milling* **155**, 40–41.

644 Raica, N. Jr., Scott, J. and Nielsen, W. (1972). The nutritional quality of irradiated foods. *Radiation Res. Rev.* **3**, 447–457.

645 Rajalakshmi, K. and Vanaja, K. (1967). Chemical and biological evaluation of the effects of fermentation on the nutritive value of foods prepared from rice and grams. *Brit. J. Nutr.* **21**, 467–473.

646 Reber, E. F., Raheja, K. and Davis, D. (1966). Wholesomeness of irradiated foods. An annotated bibliography. *Fed. Proc.* **25**, 1530–1579.

647 Salem, S. A. (1974). Effect of gamma radiation on the storage of onion used in the dehydration industry. *J. Sci. Fd. Agric.* **25**, 257–262.

648 Sheffner, A. L., Adachi, R. and Spector, H. (1957). The effect of radiation processing upon the *in vitro* digestibility and nutritional quality of proteins. *Food Res.* **22**, 455–461.

649 Shiraishi, M., Takagi, S., Tada, M. and Kawabe, S. (1974). Effect of gamma irradiation on the stability of β-carotene. *Food Sci. Tech. Abst.* **6**, 11, A 512.

650 Srinivas, H., Ananthaswamy, H. N., Vakil, U. K., and Sreenivasan, A. (1972). Effect of gamma radiation on wheat proteins. *J. Fd. Sci.* **37**, 715–719.

651 Steinkraus, K. H. and van Veen, A. G. (1971). Biochemical, nutritional and organoleptic changes occurring during production of traditional fermented foods. *In* 'Global Impacts of Applied Microbiology', 3rd. Int. Conf. Ed. Freitas, Y. M. and Fernandez, F. IBP–UNESCO Symposium.

652 Tajima, M., Sekiguchi, N. and Fujimaki, M. (1970). The amino acid content in gamma-irradiated rice. *Agric. Biol. Chem. Japan* **34**, 319–320.

653 Teixeira, A. A., Dixon, J. R. *et al.* (1969b). Computer optimization of nutrient retention in the thermal processing of conduction-heating foods. *Food Technol.* **23**, 845–850.

654 Thomas, M. H., Brenner, S., Eaton, A. and Craig, V. (1949). The effect of

electronic cooking on the nutritive value of foods. *J. Amer. Dietet. Assoc.* **25**, 39–45.

655 Thomas, P. and Janave, M. T. (1973). Polyphenol oxidase activity and browning of mango fruits induced by gamma radiation. *J. Fd. Sci.* **38**, 1149–1152.
656 Thomas, P. and Janave, M. T. (1975). Effects of gamma irradiation and storage temperature on carotenoids and ascorbic acid content of mangoes on ripening. *J. Sci. Fd. Agric.* **26**, 1503–1512.
657 Underhal, B., Nordal, J., Eggum, B. and Lunde, G. (1974). The effect of ionising radiation on the nutritional value of fish (cod) protein. *Nutr. Abstr. Rev.* **44**, No. 2138.
658 Vakil, U. K., Aravindakshan, M., Srinivas, H. *et al.* (1973). Nutritional and wholesomeness studies with irradiated foods: India's programme. Symposium on Radiation preservation of Foods (Bombay). IAEA–SM–166/12, 673.
658a Van Buren, J. P., Hackler, L. P. and Steinkraus, K. H. (1972). Solubilisation of soybean tempeh constituents during fermentation. *Cereal Chem.* **49**, 208–211.
659 Van Zante, H. J. and Johnson, S. K. (1970). Effect of electronic cooking on thiamin and riboflavin in buffered solutions. *J. Amer. Dietet. Assoc.* **56**, 133.
660 Varela, G., Urbano, G. and Barrionueva, M. (1976). Influence of irradiation and time of conservation on the nutritional value of potatoes. *Proc. 4th Internat. Cong. Fd. Sci. Technol.* Madrid. Vol. 1.
661 Walker, H. G., Lai, B., Rockwell, W. C. and Kohler, G. O. (1970). Preparation and evaluation of popped grains for feed use. *Cereal Chem.* **47**, 513–521.
662 Wilson, G. M. (1959). The treatment of meats with ionising radiations. 2. Observations on the destruction of thiamin. *J. Sci. Agric.* **10**, 295–300.
663 Wing, R. W. and Alexander, J. C. (1972). Effect of microwave heating on vitamin B_6 retention in chicken. *J. Amer. Dietet. Assoc.* **61**, 661–664.
664 Zepplin, M. and Elvehjem, C. A. (1944). Effect of refrigeration on retention of ascorbic acid in vegetables. *Food Res.* **9**, 100–111.
665 Ziporin, Z. Z., Kraybill, H. F. and Thach, H. J. (1957). Vitamin content of foods exposed to ionising radiations. *J. Nutr.* **63**, 201–209.

See also references 2, 16, 44, 45, 46, 58, 59, 80, 90, 93, 94, 95, 120, 124, 134, 140, 141, 145, 146, 233, 271, 335, 336, 385, 386, 448, 449, 455, 464, 483, 495, 515, 516, 700, 744, 745.

NUTRIENTS

Vitamins: General

666 Bender, A. E. (1971). The fate of vitamins in food processing operations. *In* 'Vitamins', 64–84. Ed. Stein, M. Churchill-Livingstone, Edinburgh.
667 Benterud, A. (1977). Vitamin losses during thermal processing. *In* 'Physical Chemical and Biological Changes in Food caused by Thermal Processing'. Ed. Høyem, T. and Kvåle, O. Appl. Sci. Pub.
668 Boas Fixsen, M. A. (1938–39). The vitamin content of human foods as affected by processes of cooking and canning. *Nutr. Abstr. Rev.* **8**, 281–307.
669 De Ritter, E. (1976). Stability characteristics of vitamins in processed foods. *Food Technol.* **30**, 48–54.

670 Glew, G., Hills, M. A. and Millross, J. (1971). Vitamins: The position now in large-scale catering. *In* 'Vitamins', 86–99. Ed. Stein, M. Churchill-Livingstone, Edinburgh.

671 Harris, R. S. (1959). Supplementation of foods with vitamins. *J. Agric. Fd. Chem.* **7**, 88–102.

672 Heierli, C. (1970). Loss of vitamins and nutritional studies. *Internat. Ztschr. Vitaminforsch.* **40**, 515–518.

673 Hewston, E. M., Dawson, E. H., Alexander, L. M. and Orent-Keiles, E. (1948). Vitamin and mineral content of certain foods as affected by home preparation. *Misc. Pub. 628, US Dept. Agric. Washington*, DC.

674 Holman, W. I. M. (1956). Distribution of vitamins within foods. *Nutr. Abstr. Rev.* **26**, 277–304.

675 Kläui, H. (1971). The functional (technical) use of vitamins. *In* 'Vitamins', 110–140. Ed. Stein, M. Churchill-Livingstone, Edinburgh.

676 Lee, C. R. and Harper, W. J. (1974). Photo-oxidation of selected vitamins (A, C & B_2) effect of packaging material. *J. Dairy Sci.* **57**, 594.

677 Mapson, L. W. (1956). Effect of processing on the vitamin content of foods. *Brit. Med. Bull.* **12**, 73–77.

678 Nagel, A. H. and Harris, R. S. (1943). Effect of restaurant cooking and service on vitamin content of foods. *J. Amer. Dietet. Assoc.* **19**, 23–25.

679 Oser, B. L., Melnick, D. and Oser, M. (1943). Influence of cooking procedure upon retention of vitamins and minerals in vegetables. *Food Res.* **8**, 115–122.

See also references 1, 2, 123, 124, 157, 170, 171, 172, 191, 418, 510, 512, 517, 519, 842, 846.

Vitamin A

680 Bauernfeind, J. C. (1974). Carotenoids and food technology. *In* 'Encyclopaedia of Food Technology', 163, Avi Publishing Co., Westport, Conn.

681 Bector, B. S. and Naranyanan, K. M. (1975). Comparative stability of unsaponifiable constituents of ghee during thermal oxidation. *Ind. J. Nutr. Dietet.* **12**, 178–180.

682 Benterud, A. *ibid*, 667.

683 Borenstein, B. and Bunnell, R. H. (1966). Carotenoids. Properties, occurrence and utilization in foods. *Adv. Fd. Res.* **15**, 195.

684 Deuel, H. J. and Greenberg, S. M. (1953). A comparison of the retention of vitamin A in margarines and butters based upon bioassays. *Food Res.* **18**, 497–503.

685 Hattiangdi, G. S. and Kanga, K. F. (1956). Heat stability of vitamin A in ghee and vanaspati. *J. Sci. Ind. Res. (India)* **15C**, 48.

686 Livingston, A. L., Knowles, R. E. and Kohler, G. O. (1970). Xanthophyll, carotene and alpha-tocopherol stability in alfalfa as affected by pilot- and industrial scale-dehydration. *U.S. Dept. Agric., Agric. Res. Serv. Tech. Bull.* No. 1414, 14.

687 Maqsood, A. S., Haque, S. A. and Khan, A. H. (1963). Stability of vitamin A in ghee and vitaminised vanaspati. *Pakist. J. Scient. Ind. Res.* **6**, 119–121.

688 Marusich, W., De Ritter, E. and Bauernfeind, J. C. (1959). Provitamin A activity and stability of β-carotene in margarine. *J. Amer. Oil Chem. Soc* **34**, 217.

689   McWeeny, D. J. (1968). Deterioration of β-carotene in certain hydrogenated fats. 1. Incidence of green discolouration during storage. 2. Products of β-carotene deterioration and nature of the green pigment. 3. Factors affecting the rate at which green discolouration occurs. *J. Sci. Fd. Agric.* **19**, 250–265.

690   Roberts, W. K. and Sell, J. L. (1963). Vitamin A destruction by nitrate *in vitro* and *in vivo. J. Animal Sci.* **22**, 1081–1085.

690a   Thompson, S. Y. (1971). *In* 'Vitamins', P. 85. Ed. Stein, M. Churchill-Livingstone, Edinburgh.

691   Wierzchowski, Z. (1956). The influence of temperature, oxygen and light on the carotene content of green forages during drying. *Nutr. Abstr. Rev.* **26**, 351.

See also references 47, 159, 212, 213, 299, 312, 320, 325, 327, 328, 329, 333, 369, 373, 375, 379, 380, 383, 384, 389, 394, 502, 508, 534, 544, 568, 571, 583, 610, 614, 649.

B vitamins

692   Arnold, A. and Elvehjem, C. A. (1939). Processing and thiamin. *Food Res.* **4**, 547–553.

693   Bendix, G. H., Heberlein, D. G., Ptak, L. R. and Clifcorn, L. E. (1951). Factors influencing the stability of thiamine during heat sterilisation. *Food Res.* **16**, 494–503.

693a   Chan, J. K. C. and Hilker, D. M. (1976). The kinetics of thiamine degradation by polyphenol derivatives catalysed by polyphenol oxidase in plant products. *Proc. 4th Internat. Cong. Fd. Sci. Technol.* Madrid. Vol. 1.

694   Dwivedi, B. K. and Arnold, R. G. (1971). Hydrogen sulphide from heat degradation of thiamin. *J. Agric. Fd. Chem.* **19**, 923.

695   Dwivedi, B. K. and Arnold, R. G. (1973a). Chemistry of thiamin degradation in food products and model systems. A review. *J. Agric. Fd. Chem.* **21**, 54–60.

696   Dwivedi, B. K. and Arnold, R. G. (1973b). Some minor volatile components from thermally degraded thiamin. *J. Fd. Sci.* **38**, 450–451.

697   Farrer, K. T. H. (1950). The thermal loss of vitamin B_1 on storage of foodstuffs. *Austral. J. Exp. Biol. Med.* **28**, 245–252.

698   Farrer, K. T. H. (1955). The thermal destruction of vitamin B_1 in foods. *Adv. Fd. Res.* **6**, 257–311.

699   Hellstrom, V. (1969). Yields of thiamine, riboflavine and niacin on baking with baking powder. *Food Sci. Tech. Abstr.* **1**, 1436; abstr. HM813.

700   Goldblith, S. A., Tannenbaum, S. R. and Wang, D. I. C. (1968). Thermal and MHz microwave energy effect on the destruction of thiamin. *Food Technol.* **22**, 1266.

701   Herbert, V. and Jacob, E. (1974). Destruction of vitamin B_{12} by ascorbic acid. *J. Amer. Dietet. Assoc.* **230**, 241–242.

702   Hermus, R. J. J. (1970). Sulphite-induced thiamine cleavage. Effect of storage and preparation of minced meat. *Nutr. Abstr. Rev.* **40**, 51.

703   Hollenbeck, C. M. and Obermeyer, H. G. (1952). Relative stability of thiamine mononitrate and thiamine hydrochloride in enriched flour. *Cereal Chem.* **29**, 82–87.

704   Kuo, J. Y. and Hilker, D. M. (1973). A fluorescent thiamin derivative formed by reacting hemin and thiamin. Effect on thiamin-deficient rats. *Nutr. Repts. Internat.* **8**, 169–174.

705   Lane, R. L., Johnson, E. and Williams, R. R. (1942). Studies of the average American diet. 1. Thiamine content. *J. Nutr.* **23**, 613–624.
706   Mason, J. B., Gibson, N. and Kodicek, E. (1973). The chemical nature of the bound nicotinic acid of wheat bran; studies of nicotinic-acid-containing macromolecules. *Brit. J. Nutr.* **30**, 297–311.
707   Mulley, E. A., Stumbo, C. R. and Hunting, W. M. (1975). Kinetics of thiamin degradation by heat. *J. Fd. Sci.* **40**, 985–988; 989–992; 993–996.
708   Orr, M. L. (1969). Pantothenic acid, vitamin B_6 and vitamin B_{12} in foods. *Home Econ. Res. Report,* No. 36, USDA, Washington, DC.
709   Porzio, M. A., Tang, N. and Hilker, D. M. (1973). Thiamin modifying properties of heme proteins from skipjack tuna, pork and beef. *J. Agric. Chem.* **21**, 308–310.
710   Press, E. and Yeagar, L. (1962). Food 'poisoning' due to sodium nicotinate. *Amer. J. publ. Hlth.* **52**, 1720–1728.
711   Rajalakshmi, R., Nanavaty, K. and Gumashta, A. (1964). Effect of cooking procedures on the free and total niacin content of certain foodstuffs. *J. Nutr. India* **1**, 276.
712   Reusser, P. (1970). Study on the photochemical inactivation of folic acid in the presence of riboflavin and its inhibition by ascorbic acid. *J. Intern. Vitaminolog.* **39**, 64. (In French.)
713   Richardson, L. R., Wilkes, S. and Ritchey, S. J. (1961a). Comparative vitamin B_6 activity of frozen, irradiated and heat-processed foods. *J. Nutr.* **73**, 363–368.
714   Srncová, W. and Davidek, J. (1972). Reaction of pyridoxal and pyridoxal-5-phosphate with proteins. *J. Fd. Sci.* **37**, 310–312.
715a Wagner-Jauregg, T. (1972). Riboflavin. II. Chemistry. *In* 'The Vitamins', Vol. 5. Ed. Sebrell, W. H., Jr. and Harris, R. S. Academic Press, New York.
716   Wendt, G. and Bernhart, F. W. (1960). The structure of a sulfur-containing compound with vitamin B_6 activity. *Arch. Biochem. Biophys.* **88**, 270–272.

See also references 9, 10, 17, 18, 19, 20, 21, 22, 23, 27, 28, 29, 30, 31, 33, 34, 40, 41, 45, 49, 50, 53, 54, 56, 57, 60, 61, 62, 63, 64, 65, 66, 69, 70, 71, 72, 74, 75, 79, 80, 81, 82, 83, 85, 86, 87, 89, 90, 92, 97, 101, 103, 151, 152, 158, 162, 163, 165, 171, 175, 176, 181, 190, 199, 200, 202a, 209, 210, 217, 220, 225, 226, 228, 234, 238, 239, 243, 244, 248, 260, 261, 266, 268, 277, 279, 280, 285, 286, 287, 292, 293, 296, 306, 386, 417, 419, 429, 440, 446, 453, 456, 464, 471, 475, 484, 485, 490, 492, 493, 502, 505, 546, 554, 556, 562, 563, 565, 571, 572, 573, 583, 587, 594, 598, 602, 610, 612, 613, 622, 638, 641, 659, 662, 663.

Folic acid

717   Bannerjee, D. K. and Chatterjea, J. B. (1964). Folic acid activity in Indian dietary articles and the effect of cooking on it. *Food Technol.* **18**, 1081–1083.
718   Colman, N., Green, R. and Metz, J. (1975). Prevention of folic acid deficiency by food fortification. II. Absorption of folic acid from fortified staple foods. *Amer. J. Clin. Nutr.* **28**, 459–464.
719   Herbert, V. (1968). Folic acid deficiency in man. *Vitamins and Hormones* **26**, 525.
720   Hurdle, A. D. F., Barton, D. and Searles, I. H. (1968). A method for measuring folate in food and its application to a hospital diet. *Amer. J. Clin. Nutr.* **21**, 1202–1207.

721 Malin, J. D. (1975). Folic acid. *World Rev. Nut. Diet.* **21**, 198–217.
722 Matoth, Y., Pinkas, A., Sroka, C. (1965). Studies on folic acid in infancy. 3. Folates in breast-fed infants and their mothers. *Amer. J. Clin. Nutr.* **16**, 356–359.
723 Taguchi, H:, Hara, K., Hasei, T. and Sanada, H. (1973). Study of folic acid content of foods. II. Loss of folates from foods by boiling. *Vitamin* **47**, 21–25; *Nutr. Abstr. Rev.* **44**, No. 7097 (1974).

See also references 164, 171, 172, 173, 175, 202a, 259, 506, 571, 584.

Vitamin C

724 Bauernfeind, J. C. and Pinkert, D. M. (1970). Food processing with added ascorbic acid. *Adv. Fd. Res.* **18**, 219.
725 Brenner, S., Wodicka, W. O. and Dunlop, S. G. (1947). Stability of ascorbic acid in various carriers. *Food Res.* **12**, 253–269.
726 Jackson, S. F., Chichester, C. O. and Joslyn, M. A. (1960). The browning of ascorbic acid. *Food Res.* **25**, 484–490.
727 Kläui, H. (1974). Technical uses of vitamin C. *In* 'Vitamin C'. Ed. Birch, G. G. and Parker, K. J. Applied Science Publishers, London.
728 Lee, S. H. and Labuza, T. P. (1975). Destruction of ascorbic acid as a function of water activity. *J. Fd. Sci.* **40**, 370–373.
729 Lopez, A., Krehl, W. A. and Good, E. (1966). Influence of time and temperature on ascorbic acid stability. *J. Amer. Dietet. Assoc.* **50**, 308–310.
730 Olliver, M. (1967). Ascorbic acid. *In* 'The Vitamins', Ed. Sebrell, W. H. and Harris, R. S. Academic Press, New York.
731 Quadri, S. F., Liang, Y. T., Seib, P. A. *et al.* (1976). Stability of L-ascorbate 2-sulphate and L-ascorbate in wheat foods and milk. *J. Fd. Sci.* **40**, 837–839.
732 Quadri, S. F., Seib, P. A. and Deyoe, C. W. (1973). Improved methods of preparing L-ascorbic acid 2-sulphate. *Carbohydrate Res.* **29**, 259.
733 Richardson, J. E. and Mayfield, H. L. (1944). Influence of sugars, fruit acids and pectin on the oxidation of ascorbic acid. *Montana State Coll. Agric. Exp. Sta. Bull.* No. 423, 20.
734 Singh, R. P., Heldman, D. R. and Kirk, J. R. (1976). Kinetics of quality degradation; ascorbic acid oxidation in infant formula during storage. *J. Fd. Sci.* **41**, 304–308.
735 Wanninger, L. A. (1972). Mathematical model predicts stability of ascorbic acid in food products. *Food Technol.* **26** (6), 42–45.
736 Wedzicha, B. L. and McWeeny, D. J. (1974). Non-enzymic browning reactions of ascorbic acid and their inhibition. The production of 3-deoxy-4-sulphopentosulose in mixtures of ascorbic acid, glycine and disulphate ion. *J. Sci. Fd. Agric.* **25**, 577–587; 589–594.
737 Zacharias, R. (1965). Ascorbic acid losses in preparation and processing of foods. *Wissenschaftl. Veröffentl. Deutsch. Gessllsch. Ernährung.* **14**, 187–205 (in German).

See also references 47, 68, 156, 165, 179a, 189, 190, 298, 302, 308, 309, 310, 311, 313, 314, 315, 316, 319, 320, 321, 322, 326, 327, 329, 330, 331, 332, 334, 337, 338, 340, 342, 343, 346, 347, 348, 349, 350, 352, 353, 354, 355, 361, 366, 367, 367a, 368, 370, 371, 374, 382, 386, 388, 393, 417, 429, 442, 446, 453, 462, 475, 478, 479, 480, 481,

482, 484, 485, 487, 488, 490, 491, 497, 499, 500, 518, 530, 556, 561, 562, 563, 568, 573, 580, 583, 585, 606, 611, 612, 615, 624, 656, 664, 701, 712, 823, 844.

Other vitamins

738   Bancher, E., Washüttl, J. and Schiffauer, R. (1973). Effect of gamma-rays on vitamin E factors in solution. 1. Tributyrin solution of alpha-tocopherol acetate and alpha-, beta-, gamma-, and delta-tocopherol. *Internat. J. Vit. and Nutr. Res.* **43**, 510–516.

739   Bancher, E., Washüttl, J. and Schiffauer, R. (1974). The effect of gamma rays on vitamin E factors in solution. 2. Tributyrin solutions of alpha-, beta-, gamma- and delta-tocotrienol. *Internat. J. Vit. and Nutr. Res.* **44**, 26–31.

740   Bunnell, R. H., Keating, J., Quaresimo, A. and Parman, G. K. (1965). Alpha-tocopherol contents of foods. *Amer. J. Clin. Nutr.* **17**, 1–10.

741   Harris, R. S. (1962). Influences of storage and processing on the retention of vitamin E in foods. *Vitamins and Hormones* **20**, 603.

742   Hogue, D. E., Proctor, J. F., Warner, R. G. and Loosli, J. K. (1962). Relation of selenium, vitamin E, and an unidentified factor to muscular dystrophy (Stiff-lamb or white-muscle disease) in the lamb. *J. Animal Sci.* **21**, 25.

743   Moore, T., Sharman, I. M. and Ward, R. J. (1957). The destruction of vitamin E in flour by chlorine dioxide. *J. Sci. Fd. Agric.* **8**, 97–104.

744   Richardson, L. R., Wilkes, S. and Ritchey, S. J. (1961b). Comparative vitamin K activity of frozen, irradiated and heat-processsed foods. *J. Nutr.* **73**, 369–373.

745   Richardson, L. R., Woodworth, P. and Coleman, S., (1956). Effect of ionizing radiations on vitamin K. *Fed. Proc.* **15**, 924–926.

746   Scheiner, J. and De Ritter, E. (1975). Biotin content of feedstuffs. *J. Agric. Fd. Chem.* **23**, 1157–1162.

747   Smith, C. L., Kelleher, J., Losowsky, M. S. and Morrish, N. (1971). The content of vitamin E in British diets. *Brit. J. Nutr.* **26**, 89.

See also references 111, 235, 247, 253, 290, 317, 502, 850.

PROTEINS

747a   Adrian, J. (1973). Aromatic substances from the Maillard reaction. *Ind. Alim. Agric.* **90**, 559.

747b   Adrian, J. (1974). Nutritional and physiological consequences of the Maillard reaction. *World Rev. Nutr. Dietet.* **19**, 71–122.

748   Adrian, J. and Fragne, R. (1973). La reaction de Maillard. Rôle des premelanoîdines sur la digestibilité azotée *in vivo* et la proteolyse *in vitro*. *Ann. Nutr. Alim.* **27**, 111–123.

749   Andrews, F., Bjorksten, J., Trenk, F. B. *et al.* (1965). The reaction of an autoxidised lipid with proteins. *J. Amer. Oil Chem. Soc.* **42**, 779.

749a   Bailey, C. J. (1974). Automated analysis of available lysine and tyrosine in foodstuffs. *J. Sci. Fd. Agric.* **25**, 1007–1014.

750   Beek, L. van, Feron, V. J. and Groot, de A. P. (1974). Nutritional effects of alkali treated soy protein in rats. *J. Nutr.* **104**, 1630–1636.

751   Bender, A. E. (1965). Loss of nutritive value of proteins through processing

and storage. *Proc. 1st Internat. Cong. Food Sci. Technol.* Vol. 3, 449–455. Gordon and Breach Publ.

752 Bender, A. E. (1965). The balancing of amino acid mixtures and proteins. *Proc. Nutr. Soc.* **24**, 190–196.

753 Bender, A. E. (1972). Processing damage to protein food: A review. *J. Fd. Technol.* **7**, 239–250.

754 Bender, A. E. (1975). Rat assay for protein quality – A reappraisal. *Proc. 9th Internat. Cong. Nutr.* Vol. 3, 310–320. Karger, Basel (1972).

755 Ben-Gera, I. and Zimmerman, G. (1972). Changes in the nitrogenous constituents of staple foods and feeds during storage. 1. Decrease in the chemical availability of lysine. *J. Fd. Sci. Technol.* **9**, 113–118.

756 Bjarnason, J. and Carpenter, K. J. (1969). Mechanisms of heat damage in proteins: models with acylated lysine units. *Brit. J. Nutr.* **23**, 859–868.

757 Bjarnason, J. and Carpenter, K. J. (1970). Mechanisms of heat damage in proteins: 2. Chemical changes in pure proteins. *Brit. J. Nutr.* **24**, 313–328.

757a Block, R. J., Cannon, P. R., Wissler, R. W. *et al.* (1946). The effects of baking and toasting on the nutritive value of protein. *Arch. Biochem.* **10**, 295–301.

758 Block, R. J. and Mitchell, H. H. (1946–1947). The correlation of the amino acid composition of proteins with their nutritive value. *Nutr. Abstr. Rev.* **16**, 249–278.

759 Boctor, A. M. and Harper, A. E. (1968). Measurement of available lysine in heated and unheated foodstuffs by chemical and biological methods. *J. Nutr.* **94**, 289–296.

760 Bohak, Z. (1964). N-epsilon-(DL-2-amino-2-carboxyethyl)-L-lysine, a new amino acid formed on alkaline treatment of proteins. *J. biol. Chem.* **239**, 2878–2887.

761 Booth, V. H. (1971). Problems in the determination of FDNB-available lysine. *J. Sci. Fd. Agric.* **22**, 658–666.

762 Boyne, A. W., Price, S. A., Rosen, G. D. and Scott, J. A. (1967). Protein quality of feedingstuffs. 4. Progress report on collaborative studies on the microbiological assay of available amino acids. *Brit. J. Nutr.* **21**, 181–206.

763 Carpenter, K. J. (1960). The estimation of available lysine in animal protein foods. *Biochem. J.* **77**, 604–610.

763a Carpenter, K. J. and Booth, V. H. (1973). Damage to lysine in food processing; its measurement and significance. *Nutr. Abstr. Rev.* **43**, 423–451.

763b Carpenter, K. J., Morgan, C. B., Lea, C. H. and Parr, L. J. (1962). Chemical and nutritional changes in stored herring meal. 3. Effect of heating at controlled moisture contents on the binding of amino acids in freeze-dried herring presscake and in related model systems. *Brit. J. Nutr.* **16**, 451–465.

764 Carpenter, K. J. and Opstvedt, J. (1976). Application of chemical and biological assay procedures for lysine in fish meals. *J. Agric. Fd. Chem.* **24**, 389–393.

765 Conkerton, E. J. and Frampton, V. L. (1959). Reaction of gossypol with free epsilon-amino groups of lysine in proteins. *Arch. Biochem. Biophys.* **81**, 130–134.

766 Cuq, J. L., Provonsal, M. P. *et al.* (1976). Effects of oxidative and alkaline treatment of food proteins on the nutritional availability of methionine and lysine. *Proc. 4th Internat. Cong. Fd. Sci. Technol.* Madrid. Vol. 1.

767 Cuq, J. L., Provansal, M. P., Guilleux, F. and Cheftel, C. (1973). Oxidation of methionine residues of casein by hydrogen peroxide. Effects on *in vitro* digestibility. *J. Fd. Sci.* **38**, 11–13.

768   Damaty, S. and Hudson, B. F. J. (1974). A secondary interaction between gossypol and cottonseed protein. *Proc. Nutr. Soc.* **34**, 49A.

769   De Groot, A. P. and Slump, P. (1969). Effects of severe alkali treatment of proteins on amino acid composition and nutritive value. *J. Nutr.* **98**, 45–56.

770   Desai, I. D. and Tappel, A. L. (1963). Damage to proteins by peroxidised lipids. *J. Lipid Res.* **4**, 204.

771   Devik, O. G. (1967). Formation of *N*-nitrosamines by the Maillard reaction. *Acta. Chem. Scand.* **21**, 2302–2303.

772   Donoso, G., Lewis, O. A. M., Miller, D. S. and Payne, P. R. (1962). Effect of heat treatment on the nutritive value of proteins; Chemical and balance studies. *J. Sci. Fd. Agric.* **13**, 192–196.

773   Dümmer, H. W. (1971). Availability of amino acids in heat damaged protein. *Nutr. Abst. Rev.* **41**, No. 5250.

774   Eldred, N. R. and Rodney, G. (1946). The effect of proteolytic enzymes on raw and heated casein. *J. biol. Chem.* **162**, 261–265.

775   Eichner, K. and Karel, M. (1972). The influence of water content and water activity on the sugar-amino browning reaction in model systems under various conditions. *J. Agric. Fd. Chem.* **20**, 218–223.

776   Ellinger, G. M. and Palmer, R. (1969). The biological availability of methionine sulfoxide. *Proc. Nutr. Soc.* **28**, 42A.

777   Ellis, G. P. (1959). The Maillard reaction. *Adv. Carbohydrate Chem.* **14**, 63–134.

778   El Miladi, S. S., Gould, W. A. and Clements, R. L. (1969). Heat processing effect on starch, sugars and proteins, amino acids and organic acids of tomato juice. *Food Technol.* **23**, 691–693.

779   Ershoff, B. H. and Rucker, P. G. (1969). Nutritive value of 1, 2-dichloro-ethane-extracted FPC. *J. Fd. Sci.* **34**, 355–359.

779a   Evans, R. J. and Butts, H. A. (1948). Studies on the heat inactivation of lysine in soy bean oil meal. *J. biol. Chem.* **175**, 15–20.

779b   Evans, R. J. and Butts, H. A. (1949). Studies on the heat inactivation of methionine in soy bean oil meal. *J. biol. Chem.* **178**, 543-548.

780   FAO (1970). FAO Nutritional Studies No. 24, Amino Acid Content of Foods and Biological Data on Proteins. (FAO, Rome.)

781   Ferretti, A. and Flanagan, V. P. (1971). The lactose-casein (Maillard) browning system: volatile compounds. *J. Agric. Fd. Chem.* **19**, 245–249.

782   Finot, P. A. (1973). Non-enzymic browning. *In* 'Proteins in Human Nutrition', 501–514. Ed. Porter, J. W. G. and Rolls, B. A. Academic Press, London.

783   Finot, P. A. and Mauron, J. (1972). Damage to lysine by the Maillard reaction. *Helvetica Chimica Acta* **55**, 1153–1164.

784   Fixsen, M. A. B. (1934). The biological value of protein in nutrition. *Nutr. Abstr. Rev.* **4**, 447–459.

785   Finot, P. A., Viani, R. and Mauron, J. (1968). Identification of a new lysine derivative obtained upon acid hydrolysis of heated milk. *Experimentia* **24**, 1097–1099.

786   Folk, J. E. (1956). The influence of the lysine-glucose reaction on enzymatic digestion. *Arch. Biochem. Biophys.* **64**, 6-18.

787   Ford, J. E. (1962). A microbiological method for assessing the nutritional value of proteins. *Brit. J. Nutr.* **16**, 409–425.

788   Ford, J. E. and Shorrock, C. (1971). Metabolism of heat damaged protein in the rat. *Brit. J. Nutr.* **26**, 311–322.

789   Greaves, E. O., Morgan, A. F. and Loveen, M. K. (1938). The effect of amino acid supplementation and of variations in temperature and duration of heating upon the biological value of heated casein. *J. Nutr.* **16**, 115–128.

790   Griswold, R. M. (1951). Effect of heat on nutritive value of proteins. *J. Amer. Dietet. Assoc.* **27**, 85–93.

791   Halevy, S. and Guggenheim, K. (1953). The biological availability of heated wheat gluten-glucose mixtures. *Arch. Biochem. Biophys.* **44**, 211–217.

792   Hayase, F., Kato, H. and Fujimaki, M. (1975). Racemization of amino acid residues in proteins and poly (L-amino acids) during roasting. *J. Agric. Fd. Chem.* **23**, 491–494.

793   Henry, K. M. and Kon, S. K. (1950). Effect of reaction with glucose on the nutritional value of casein. *Biochem. Biophys. Acta.* **5**, 455.

794   Herz, W. J. and Shallenberger, R. S. (1960). Some aromas produced by simple amino acid-sugar reactions. *Food Res.* **25**, 491–494.

795   Hodge, J. E. (1953). The chemistry of browning reactions. *J. Agr. Fd. Chem.* **1**, 928–943.

796   Horn, M. J., Lichtenstein, H. and Womack, M. (1968). A methionine-fructose compound and its availability to micro-organisms and rats. *J. Agric. Fd. Chem.* **16**, 741–745.

797   Hussein, L. A. (1974). Comparison of methods for the determination of available lysine value in animal protein concentrations. *J. Sci. Fd. Agric.* **25**, 117–120.

798   Jones, L. A. and Smith, F. H. (1975). Effects of free and bound gossypol on the absorption of L-(14-C) lysine, L-(14-C) methionine and L-(14-C) valine from the rat small intestine. *J. Agric. Fd. Chem.* **23**, 647–653.

799   Karel, M., Schaich, K. and Roy, R. B. (1975). Interaction of peroxidising methyl linoleate with some proteins and amino acids. *J. Agric. Fd. Chem.* **23**, 159–163.

800   Lakin, A. L. (1973). Evaluation of protein quality by dye-binding procedures, pp. 179–194. *In* 'Proteins in Human Nutrition', Ed. Porter, J. W. G. and Rolls, B. A. Academic Press, London.

801   Lea, C. H. and Hannan, R. S. (1949). Studies on the reaction between protein and reducing sugars in the 'dry' state. I. The effect of activity of water, of pH and of temperature on the primary reaction between casein and glucose. *Biochem. Biophys. Acta* **3**, 313.

802   Lea, C. H. and Hannan, R. S. (1950). Studies on the reaction between protein and reducing sugars in the 'dry' state. II. Further observations on the formation of the casein-glucose complex. *Biochem. Biophys. Acta* **4**, 518.

803   Lee, C. M., Chichester, C. O. and Lee, T-C. (1976). Physiological consequences of browned food products. *Proc. 4th Internat. Cong. Fd. Sci. Technol.* Madrid. Vol. 1.

804   Lowry, J. R. and Thiessen, R. (1950). Studies on the nutritive impairment of proteins heated with carbohydrates. II. *In vitro* digestion studies. *Arch. Biochem.* **25**, 148–156.

805   Mader, I. J., Schroeder, L. J. and Smith, A. H. (1949). The effect of carbohydrate on the nutritive value of heated lactalbumin. *J. Nutr.* **39**, 341–355.

806   McKinney, L. L., Weakley, F. B., Eldridge, A. C. *et al.* (1957). S-(dichloro vinyl)-L-cysteine; an agent causing fatal aplastic anaemia in calves. *J. Amer. Chem. Soc.* **79**, 3932–3933.

807   McWeeny, D. J., Knowles, M. E. and Hearne, J. F. (1974). The chemistry of

non-enzymic browning in foods and its control by sulphites. *J. Sci. Fd. Agric.* **25**, 735–746.

808 Mauron, J. (1961). The concept of amino acid availability and its bearing on protein evaluation. *In* 'Progress in Meeting Protein Needs of Infants and Preschool Children'. Nat. Acad. Sci. Washington, U.S.A. N.R.C. Publ. 813.

809 Mauron, J. (1976). The analytical, nutritional and toxicological implications of protein food processing. *Proc. 4th Internat. Cong. Fd. Sci. Technol.* Madrid. Vol. 1.

810 Melnick, D., Oser, B. L. and Weiss, S. (1946). Rate of enzyme digestion of proteins as a factor in nutrition. *Science, N.Y.* **103**, 326–329.

811 Miller, D. S. (1970). The nutritional evaluation of protein supplements to diets. *In* 'Evaluation of Novel Protein Products'. Ed. Bender, A. E., Kihlberg, R., Löfqvist, B. and Munck, L. Pergamon Press.

812 Morgan, A. F. (1931). the effect of heat upon the biological value of cereal proteins and casein. *J. biol. Chem.* **90**, 771–792.

813 Narayan, K. A. and Kummerow, F. A. (1963). Factors influencing the formation of complexes between oxidised lipids and proteins. *J. Amer. Oil Chem. Soc.* **40**, 339.

814 Nutr. Rev. (1976). Processed protein foods and lysinoalanine. *Nutr. Rev.* **34**, 120–122.

815 Ory, L. R. and St. Angelo, A. J. (1975). Symposium on effects of oxidised lipids on food proteins and flavour. *J. Agric. Fd. Chem.* **23**, 125–176.

816 Pieniazek, D., Rakowska, M. and Kunachowicz, H. (1975). The participation of methionine and cysteine in the formation of bonds resistant to the action of proteolytic enzymes in heated casein. *Brit. J. Nutr.* **34**, 163–173.

817 Pieniazek, D., Rakowska, M., Szkilladziowa, W. and Grabarek, Z. (1975). Estimation of available methionine and cystine in proteins of food products by *in vivo* and *in vitro* methods. *Brit. J. Nutr.* **34**, 175–190.

818 Porter, J. W. G. and Rolls, B. A. (1971). Some aspects of the digestion of proteins. *Proc. Nutr. Soc.* **30**, 17–24.

819 Pronczuk, A., Pawlowska, D. and Bartnick, J. (1973). Effect of heat treatment on the digestibility and utilisation of protein. *Nutr. Metab.* **15**, 171–180.

820 Provansal, M. M. P., Cuq, A. J.-L. Cheftel, J.-C. (1975). Chemical and nutritional modifications of sunflower proteins due to alkaline processing. Formation of amino acid cross-links and isomerisation of lysine residues. *J. Agric. Fd. Chem.* **23**, 938–943.

821 Pusztai, A. (1967). Trypsin inhibitors of plant origin, their chemistry and potential role in animal nutrition. *Nutr. Abstr. Rev.* **37**, 1–9.

823 Ranganna, S. and Setty, L. (1968). Non-enzymic discolouration in dried cabbage. Ascorbic acid – amino acid interaction. *J. Agric. Fd. Chem.* **16**, 529–533.

824 Reynolds, T. M. (1963). Chemistry of nonenzymic browning. 1. *Adv. Fd. Res.* **12**, 1–52.

825 Rice, E. E. and Beuk, J. F. (1953). The effect of heat on the nutritive value of proteins. *Adv. Fd. Res.* **4**, 233.

826 Reynolds, T. M. (1965). Chemistry of nonenzymic browning. 2. *Adv. Fd. Res.* **14**, 168–228.

827 Roubal, W. J. (1971). Free radicals, malonaldehyde and protein damage in lipid-protein systems. *Lipids* **6**, 62.

828 Stadtman, E. R. (1948). Nonenzymatic browning in fruit products. *Adv. Fd. Res.* **1**, 325.

829   Sternberg, M., Kim, C. Y. and Schwende, F. J. (1975). Lysinoalanine; presence in foods and food ingredients. *Science* **190**, 992–994.
829a Tanaka, M., Amaya, J., Lee, T.-C. and Chichester, C. O. (1977). The effects of the browning reaction on the quality of protein. *Proc. 4th Internat. Cong. Fd. Sci. Technol.* Madrid. Vol. 1.
830   Tannenbaum, S. R., Barth, H. and Le Roux, J. P. (1969). Loss of methionine in casein during storage with autoxidising methyl linoleate. *J. Agric. Fd. Chem.* **17**, 1353.
831   Tappel, A. L. (1955). *In vitro* copolymerisation of oxidised fats with protein. *Arch. Biochem. Biophys.* **54**, 266–280.
832   Tarr, H. L. A. (1954). The Maillard reaction in flesh foods. *Food Technol.* **8**, 15–19,
833   Underwood, J. C., Lento, H. G. and Willits, C. O. (1959). Browning of sugar solutions. 3. Effects of pH on the colour produced in dilute glucose solutions containing amino acids with amino groups in different position in the molecule. *Food Res.* **24**, 181–184.
834   Valle-Riestra, J. and Barnes, R. H. (1970). Digestion of heat damaged egg albumin by the rat. *J. Nutr.* **100**, 873–882.
835   Van Beek, L., Feron, V. J. and De Groot, A. P. (1974). Nutritional effects of alkali-treated soyprotein in rats. *J. Nutr.* **104**, 1630–1636.
836   Varma, T. N. R. (1967). Protein lipid interaction affecting the quality of protein foods. *J. Fd. Sci. Technol.* **4**, 12–13.
837   Warmbier, H. C., Schnickels, R. A. and Labuza, T. P. (1976). Non-enzymatic browning kinetics in an intermediate moisture system; effect of glucose to lysine ratio. *J. Fd. Sci.* **41**, 981–983.
838   Wilson, R. A. (1975). A Review of thermally produced imitation meat flavours. *J. Agric. Fd. Chem.* **23**, 1032–1037.
839   Womack, M., Bodwell, C. E. and Vaughan, D. A. (1974). Estimation of the changes in the availability of each individual essential amino acid in food proteins. *J. Fd. Sci.* **39**, 490–493.
840   Woodard, J. C. and Short, D. D. (1973). Toxicity of alkali-treated soyprotein in rats. *J. Nutr.* **103**, 569–574.

See also references 4, 5, 6, 7, 15, 16, 23, 24, 25, 26, 36, 43, 58, 59, 77, 88, 94, 102, 106, 107, 108, 112, 113, 114, 115, 117, 119, 121, 122, 127, 128, 129, 130, 131, 132, 133, 134, 135, 136, 138, 142, 143, 148, 149, 150, 155, 160, 161, 166, 167, 168, 169, 183, 184, 185, 187, 197, 203, 211, 214, 215, 221, 222, 227, 229, 230, 231, 236, 237, 245, 246, 249, 250, 251, 252, 256, 257, 258, 265, 267, 269, 270, 271, 272, 273, 276, 277, 280, 282, 283, 284, 288, 289, 294, 295, 297, 301, 303, 304, 305, 323, 395, 396, 397, 398, 399, 404, 410, 411, 416, 426, 431, 432, 438, 439, 443, 451, 452, 454, 467, 472, 474, 475, 503, 504, 509, 533, 570.

MINERAL SALTS AND CARBOHYDRATES

841   Fagerson, I. S. (1969). Thermal degradation of carbohydrates. *J. Agric. Fd. Chem.* **17**, 747–750.
842   Hein, R. E. and Hutchings, I. J. (1971). Influence of processing on vitamin-mineral content and biological availability in processed foods. *In* 'Symposium on Vitamins and Minerals in Processed Foods'. Am. Med. Assn.

Council on Foods and Nutrition and Food Industry Liaison Committee, New Orleans.

843	Kuhajek, E. J. and Fiedelman, H. W. (1973). Nutritional iodine in processed foods. *Food Technol.* **27**, 52–53.

844	Kunkel, W. (1966). Nutrient losses in the preparation of foods by automatically operated large-scale cooking equipment. I. Statement of the problem and losses of total vitamin C. II. Minerals. *Nutr. Abstr. Rev.* **36**, No. 541, 2143. (In German.)

845	Saito, Y. (1969). An experimental study of the changes in iron during cooking processes of daily foods. *J. Jap. Soc. Fd. Nutr.* **22**, 518–525; 526–530. *Nutr. Abst. Rev.* 1970, **40**, Nos. 6961, 6962.

846	Schroeder, H. A. (1971). Losses of vitamins and trace minerals from processing and preservation of foods. *Amer. J. Clin. Nutr.* **24**, 562–573.

847	Sinar, L. J. and Mason, M. (1975). Effect of rinsing and heating in water. Sodium in four canned vegetables. *J. Amer. Dietet. Assoc.* **66**, 155–157.

848	Theuer, R. C. *et al.* (1971). Effect of processing on availability of iron salts in liquid infant formula products, experimental soy isolate formulas. *J. Agric. Fd. Chem.* **19**, 555–558.

See also references 2, 47, 85, 104, 118, 349, 350, 433, 465, 673, 679.

FATS

849	Alfin-Slater, R. B., Auerbach, S. and Aftergood, L. (1959). Nutritional evaluation of some heated oils. *J. Amer. Oil Chem. Soc.* **36**, 638–641.

850	Alfin-Slater, R. B., Morris, R. B., Aftergood, L. and Melnick, D. (1969). Dietary fat composition and tocopherol requirement. II. Nutritional status of heated and unheated vegetable oils of different ratios of unsaturated fatty acids and vitamin E. *J. Amer. Oil Chem. Soc.* **46**, 657–661.

851	Artman, N. R. (1969). The chemical and biological properties of heated and oxidised fats. *Adv. Lipid Res.* **7**, 245–330.

852	Balnave, D. (1968). Influence of dietary linoleic acid on egg fatty acid composition in hens deficient in essential fatty acids. *J. Sci. Fd. Agric.* **19**, 266–269.

853	Bennion, M. and Park, R. L. (1968). Changes in frying fats with different foods. *J. Amer. Dietet. Assoc.* **52**, 308–312.

854	Carlin, G. T., Hopper, R. P. and Rockwood, B. N. (1954). Some factors affecting the decomposition of frying fats. *Food Technol.* **8**, 161–165.

855	Chiphault, J. R. and Mizuno, G. R. (1966). Effect of ionising radiations on stability of fats. *J. Agric. Fd. Chem.* **14**, 225–229.

856	Cook, L. J., Scott, T. W., Faichney, G. J. and Davies, H. L. (1972). Fatty acids interrelationships in plasma, liver, muscle and adipose tissues of cattle fed safflower oil protected from ruminal hydrogenation. *Lipids* **7**, 83–89.

857	Cook, L. J., Scott, T. W., Ferguson, K. A. and McDonald, I. W. (1970). Production of polyunsaturated ruminant body fats. *Nature, Lond.* **228**, 178–179.

858	Crampton, E. W., Common, R. H., Farmer, F. A., Wells, A. F. and Crawford, D. (1953). Studies to determine the nature of the damage to the nutritive value of some vegetables from heat treatment. III. The segregation of toxic and non-toxic material from the esters of heat polymerized linseed oil by distillation and by urea adduct formation. *J. Nutr.* **49**, 333–346.

859 Fleischman, A. I., Florin, A., Fitzgerald, J., Caldwell, A. B. and Eastwood, G. (1963). Studies on cooking fats and oils. *J. Amer. Dietet. Assoc.* **42**, 394–398.

860 Friedman, L., Horwitz, W., Shue, G. M. and Firestone, D. (1961). Heated fats. II. The nutritive properties of heated cottonseed oil and of heated cottonseed oil fractions. *J. Nutr.* **73**, 85–93.

861 Gurr, M. I. (1970). Biosynthesis of unsaturated fatty acids. *Chem. Indust.* 1393–1407.

862 Harkins, R. W. and Sarrett, H. P. (1968). Medium chain triglycerides. *J. Amer. med. Assoc.* **203**, 272–274.

863 Heidelbaugh, N. D., Yeh, C. P. and Karel, M. (1971). Effects of model system composition on autoxidation of methyl linoleate. *J. Agric. Fd. Chem.* **19**, 140.

864 Johnson, O. C. (1961). Studies on the nutritional and physiological effects of theramally oxidised oils. *J. Amer. Oil Chem. Soc.* **38**, 99.

865 Kaunitz, H. R., Johnson, R. E. and Pegus, L. (1965). A long term nutritional study with fresh and mildly oxidised vegetable and animal fats. *J. Amer. Oil Chem. Soc.* **42**, 770–774.

866 Kilgore, L. and Bailey, M. (1970). Degradation of linoleic acid during potato frying. *J. Amer. Dietet. Assoc.* **56**, 130–132.

867 Kilgore, L. and Luker, N. D. (1964). Fatty acid components of fried foods and fats used for frying. *J. Amer. Oil Chem. Soc.* **41**, 496–500.

868 Kilgore, L. and Windham, F. (1973). Degradation of linoleic acid in deep-fried potatoes. *J. Amer. Dietet. Assoc.* **63**, 525–527.

869 Labuza, T. P. (1971). Kinetics of lipid oxidation in foods. *Crit. Rev. Food Tech.* **2**, 355–405.

870 Langlois, G. (1967). Margarine and shortenings. *Rep. Progr. Appl. Chem.* **52**, 446–449.

871 Lee, W. T. and Dawson, L. E. (1973). Chicken lipid changes during cooking in fresh and re-used cooking oil. *J. Fd. Sci.* **38**, 1232–1237.

872 Marcuse, R. (1965). Fat oxidation as a problem in modern food preservation. *4th Fat, Oil Chem. Scand. Symp.* 191–215. (*Chem. Abstr.* **70**, 214; abstr. 36452, 1969.)

873 Melnick, D. (1957). Nutritional quality of frying fats in commercial use. *J. Amer. Oil. Chem. Soc.* **34**, 578–582.

874 Moran, D. P. J. (1968). Margarine and shortenings. *Rep. Progr. Appl. Chem.* **53**, 452–456.

875 Perkins, E. G. (1960). Nutritional and chemical changes occurring in heated fats: A review. *Food Technol.* **14**, 508–514.

876 Phillips, J. A. and Vail, G. E. (1967). Effect of heat on fatty acids. *J. Amer. Dietet. Assoc.* **50**, 116–121.

877 Poling, C. E., Warner, W. D., Mone, P. E. and Rice, E. E. (1960). The nutritional value of fats after use in commercial deep-fat frying. *J. Nutr.* **72**, 109–120.

878 Schultz, H. W., Day, E. A. and Sinnhuber, R. D. (Ed.) (1962). 'Lipids and their Oxidation'. Avi Publishing Co., Westport, Conn.

879 Scott, T. W., Cook, L. J., Ferguson, K. A. *et al.* (1970). Production of polyunsaturated milk fat in domestic ruminants. *Austr. J. Sci.* **32**, 291–293.

880 Standal, B. R., Bassett, D. R., Policar, P. B. and Thom, M. (1970). Fatty

acids, cholesterol and proximate analyses of some ready-to-eat foods. *J. Amer. Dietet. Assoc.* **56**, 392–396.
881 Wishner, L. A. and Keeney, M. (1965). Formation of carbonyl compounds during frying. *J. Amer. Oil Chem. Soc.* **42**, 776–778.
882 Zirlin, A. and Karel, M. (1969). Oxidation effects in a freeze-dried gelatin-methyl linoleate system. *J. Fd. Sci.* **34**, 160–164.

See also references 14, 26, 46, 67, 99, 100, 105, 137, 145, 146, 153, 198, 216, 218, 235, 242, 278, 280, 291, 399, 681, 684, 685, 687, 688, 689, 770, 799, 815, 831, 923.

REVIEW ARTICLES AND UNCLASSIFIED PAPERS

883 Bender, A. E. (1966). Nutritional effects of food processing. *J. Fd. Technol.* **1**, 261–289.
884 Berk, Z. (1970). Processing and storage damage to the nutritional value of foods, 189–191. *Proc. 3rd Internat. Congr. Food Sci. Technol.*
885 Bookwalter, G. N., Moser, H. A. *et al.* (1968). Storage stability of blended food products, formula No. 2: A corn-soy-milk food supplement. *Food Technol.* **22**, 1581–1584.
886 Campbell, J. A. and Morrison, A. B. (1966). Nutritional impact of modern food processing. *Fed. Proc.* **25**, 130–136.
887 Catering Research Unit (1970). An experiment in hospital catering using the cook/freeze system. University of Leeds, England.
888 Cecil, S. R. and Woodroof, J. G. (1962). Long-term storage of military rations. Quartermaster Food and Container Institute, Chicago.
889 Chandrasekhara, M. R., Ramanatham, G., and Rao, G. R. *et al.* (1964). Infant food based on coconut protein, groundnut protein isolate and skim milk powder. 1. Preparation, chemical composition and shelf-life. *J. Sci. Fd. Agric.* **15**, 839–841.
890 Chichester, C. O. (1973). Nutrition in Food Processing. *World Rev. Nutr. Dietet.* **16**, 318–333.
891 Daniels, R. W. (1974). Handbook No. 8 and Nutritional Labelling. *Food Technol.* **28**, 46.
892 Ford, J. E. (1973). Some effects of processing on nutritional value. *In* 'Proteins in Human Nutrition', 515–529. Ed. Porter, J. W. G. and Rolls, B. A. Academic Press, London.
893 Harjes, C. F. and Smith, R. J. (1970). Nutritive analysis of frozen fully cooked institutional foods. *Food Technol.* **24**, 989.
894 Harris, R. S. and Karmas, E. (1975). 'Nutritional Evaluation of Food Processing', 2nd Edn. Avi Publishing Co., Westport, Conn.
895 Harris, R. S. and von Loesecke, H. (1960). 'Nutritional Evaluation of Food Processing'. Wiley, Chichester.
896 Head, M. K. (1974). Nutrient losses in institutional food handling. *J. Amer. Dietet. Assoc.* **65**, 423–427.
897 Hearne, J. F. (1964). Long-term storage of foods. *Food Technol.* **18** (3), 60–65.
898 Hellendoorn, E. W., de Groot, A. P., van der Mijlldekker, L. P., Slump, P. and Willems, J. J. L. (1971). Effect of heat sterilisation and prolonged storage. *J. Amer. Dietet. Assoc.* **58**, 434–441.

899   Hodge, J. E. (1967). Symposium on Foods. 'The Chemistry and Physiology of Flavours'. Chap. 12. Ed. Schultz, H. W. Avi Publishing Co., Westport, Conn.
900   Hollingsworth, D. F. (1970). Effects of some new production and processing methods on nutritive values. *J. Amer. Dietet. Assoc.* **57**, 246–249.
901   IFT (1974). Effects of processing on nutritive value. Scientific status summary Institute of Food Technology. *Food Technol.* **28**, 78–81.
902   Kramer, A. (1974). Storage retention of nutrients. *Food Technol.* **28**, 50–60.
903   Lachance, P. A., Ranadive, A. S. and Matas, J. (1972). Effects of reheating convenience foods. *Food Technol.* **27**, 36–38.
904   Lang, K. (1970). Influence of cooking on foodstuffs. *World Rev. Nutr. Dietet.* **12**, 267–317.
905   Lepkovsky, S. (1953). Nutritional stress factors and food processing. *Adv. Fd. Res.* **4**, 105.
906   Liener, I. E. (1974). Phyto-hemagglutinins: their nutritional significance. *J. Agric. Fd. Chem.* **22**, 17–22.
907   Liener, I. E. and Kakade, M. L. (1969). Protease Inhibitors. *In* 'Toxic Constituents of Plant Foodstuffs', 7. Ed. Liener, I. E. Academic Press, New York.
908   Lund, D. B. *et al.* (1973). Symposium: Effects of processing, storage and handling on nutrient retention in foods. *Food Technol.* **27**, No. 1, 16–38; 51.
909   McCance, R. A. and Widdowson, E. M. (1960). The composition of foods. Med. Res. Counc. Spec. Rep. Ser. No. 297 (HMSO, London).
910   McWeeny, D. J. (1968). Reactions in food systems. Negative temperature coefficients and other abnormal temperature effects. *J. Fd. Technol.* **3**, 15–30.
911   Ministry of Agriculture, Fisheries and Food (1973). Household Food Consumption and Expenditure (1971). Annual Report of the National Food Survey Committee. HMSO, London.
912   Murphy, E. W., Criner, P. E. and Gray, B. C. (1975). Comparisons of methods for calculating retention of nutrients in cooked foods. *J. Agric. Fd. Chem.* **23**, 1153–1157.
913   Murphy, E. W., Watt, B. K. and Rizek, R. L. (1973). Tables of food composition; availability, uses and limitations. *Food Technol.* **27**, 40–51.
913a Nat. Res. Council (1961). 'Progress in Meeting Protein Needs of Infants and Preschool Children', Nat. Acad. Sci. Washington, U.S.A. N.R.C. Publ. 813.
914   Nesheim, R. O. (1974). Nutrient changes in food processing; A current review. *Federation Proc.* **33**, 2267–2269.
915   Nutrition Reviews (1975). The effects of food processing on nutritional values (Scientific Status Summary of Institute of Food Technologists' Panel). *Nutr. Rev.* **33**, 123–126.
916   Pinsent, B. R. W. (1970). Food and health. Future problems for the food manufacturer. *Commun. Hlth* **1**, 198–205.
917   Platt, B. S., Eddy, T. P., Pellett, P. L. (1963). 'Food in Hospitals'. Oxford University Press, London.
918   Sabry, Z. I. (1968). The nutritional consequences of developments in food processing. *Can. J. Pub. Health* **59**, 471–474.
919   Southgate, D. A. T. (1974). 'Guide Lines for the preparation of Tables of Food Composition'. S. Karger, Basel.
920   Spengler, M. (1971). Effect of different preservation treatments on nutritional value. *Industrielle Obst-und Gemüseverwertung* **56**, 163–164.
921   U.S. Fish and Wild Life Service, Dept. of Interior (1955). Compilation of laboratory data 'Yields and Losses in Preparation of Foods'. Mimeo.

ENRICHMENT

922   Brooke, C. L. (1968). Enrichment and fortification of cereals and cereal products with vitamins and minerals. *J. Agric. Fd. Chem.* **16**, 163–167.

923   Coulter, S. T. and Thomas, E. L. (1968). Enrichment and fortification of dairy products and margarine. *J. Agric. Fd. Chem.* **16**, 158–162.

924   Council on Foods and Nutrition (1973). Improvement of the nutritive quality of foods. *J. Amer. Med. Assoc.* **225**, 1116–1118.

925   Darby, W. J. and Hambraeus, L. (1975). Proposed nutritional guidelines for utilization of industrially produced nutrients. *Naringsforskning. Arg.* **19**, 113–120.

926   Uhl, E. (1957). Principles of enrichment of foods. *Inter. Rev. Vitamin-Res.* Vol. XXVIII, 1/2, 168–190.

927   Filer, L. J. (1968). Enrichment of special dietary food products. *J. Agric. Fd. Chem.* **16**, 184–189.

928   Harris, R. S. (1959). Attitudes and approaches to supplementation of foods with nutrients. *J. Agric. Fd. Chem.* **7**, 88–102.

929   Harris, R. S. (1968). Attitudes and approaches to supplementation of foods with nutrients. *J. Agric. Fd. Chem.* **16**, 149–152.

930   LaChance, P. A. (1970). Nutrification, a new nutritional concept. *Food Technol.* **24**, 100.

931   Lindsey, D. R. (1970). Nutritional consideration in foods. *Food Drug Cos. law J.* **25**, 38–42.

932   Menden, E. and Cremer, H. D. (1958, 1959). Improving nutritive value, special reference to enrichment. *Food Manuf.* July, Aug., Sept., Oct., Nov. (1958). Feb., Mar. (1959).

933   Mitsuda, H. (1969). New approaches to amino acid and vitamin enrichment in Japan. Protein enriched cereal foods for world needs. *J. Amer. Assoc. Cereal Chem. St. Paul.* 208–219.

934   Navia, J. M. (1968). Enrichment of sugar and sugar products. *J. Agric. Fd. Chem.* **16**, 172–176.

935   Russell, M. W., (1956). A brief history of the enrichment of flour and bread. *J. Amer. Med. Assoc.* **162**, 1539–1541.

936   Jones, D. B., Fraps, G. S. *et al.* (1943). *Bull, Nat. Res. Council, Reprint & Circular Series 116.*

937   Fraps, G. S. and Kemmerer, A. R. (1937). *Texas Agr. Expt. Sta. Bull. No. 557.*

Subject Index